正しく診断するための
診療英会話

Natural Hospital Conversations

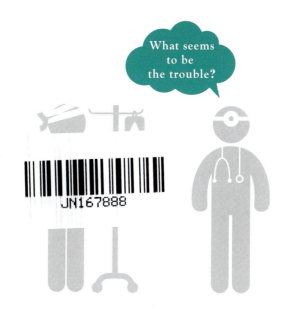

医学博士 整形外科医
バリー・ブラム＝監修

弘前大学大学院医学研究科 特任准教授
バーマン・シャーリー・J＝著

ナツメ社

はじめに

読者の皆様へ

　本書を選んでいただきありがとうございます。本書のPART 1とPART 2は全く異なった観点で構成されています。

　PART 1は、典型的な日本の病院で繰り広げられる日常のやりとりを日本人の視点から提供しています。新規の外国人の患者さんと何か会話をするときに参照するのに、PART 1は格好の入門書です。録音された日本語と英語の会話を交互に聞くことで、典型的な病院でのやりとりに精通されることでしょう。

　PART 2は、各診療科で日々繰り広げられる数多くの病状に関わる英語表現を、異文化の観点で紹介しています。PART 2によって、医療の専門家と患者さんとの間で取り交わされる他に類を見ない実践的な会話を習得されることでしょう。

　本書に登場する外国人の患者さんは、日本在住の平均的な外国人で、多くが病状に精通しています。医療従事者の中には留学や海外勤務の経験を持つ人も多いので、日本人を対象とする患者のケアとの文化的な相違点は想像に難くないでしょうが、こうした外国人の患者さんが、本編を通じて随所で使っているのは、英語の医療書で扱われている用語ではなく「lay terms（一般用語）」です。

　lay terms（一般用語）は日本の医療専門家にとって注目すべき有益な分野です。興味深いのは、英語で使われているlay termsの多くの状況が、日本語でもlay termsとして用いられていることです。たとえば、日本人は一般に、「肩関節周囲炎（専門用語）」ではなく「四十肩（一般用語）」が普及しています。同じ症状については、英語でも専門用語ではなく、「frozen shoulder（凍結肩）」という一般用語が普及しています。そうかと思うと、日本ではアレルギーの症状を説明するとき、「アレルギー鼻炎（専門用語）」を用います。英語でも一般の患者さんが専門用語で病状を説明することがあります。つまり普及している専門用語もあれば、普及していない専門用語もあるわけです。本書では、英語圏の患者さんと医師との間で今日よく用いられる会話例を多数掲載しています。

　私は弘前大学医学部医学科の医療英語コースにおいて、こうした用語を教材として作成しましたが、学生たちは一般用語と専門用語の対比に触れ大いに刺激を受けています。本書を通じてより多くの読者の皆様に教材を提供できることをうれしく思います。本書が皆様のより発展的な学習の手助けとなれば幸いです。

　本書の執筆にあたり、監修を快諾し的確なアドバイスをくださったバリー・ブラム先生、そして編集のコーディネーションや助言をいただいた（有）ジャパン・ランゲージ・フォーラムの小林裕子さん、（株）シー・レップスの飯尾美子さん、ナツメ出版企画（株）の遠藤やよいさんにこの場を借りて御礼申し上げます。

2016年5月1日
バーマン・シャーリー・J

監修のことば

I am honored to serve as Editorial Supervisor for this medical conversation book. The author, Shari Berman, has been a colleague and friend for many years. She is a brilliant linguist who has mastered many languages out of sheer interest in effective communication.

I was profoundly impressed by the scope, the depth and the accuracy of her dialogs. Bridging the communication gap between a patient and a doctor coming from different backgrounds is critically important. Ms. Berman's book is designed precisely for this purpose. Her skillful preparation of the material here should enable the Japanese medical professional to communicate with his or her English speaking patients accurately and comfortably, even with patients who speak idiomatically and not just according to the dictionaries.
Aloha,

Barry Blum, MD

本書に監修として参画できたことを光栄に思います。著者のシャーリー・バーマンは、私の長年にわたる仕事仲間であり友人です。彼女は才能ある言語学者で、効果的なコミュニケーションへの純粋な興味から多言語を習得してきました。

私は彼女が執筆した本書の会話が持つ幅広さ・奥深さに深く感銘を受けました。さまざまな経歴を持った患者と医師の間のコミュニケーションギャップを埋めることは極めて重要です。本書はまさしくこうした目的で作られています。長年の経験に基づいて構想された本書を学習すれば、日本人の医療従事者が英語圏の患者と、たとえ彼らが一般的な話し言葉を使ったとしても、正確かつ無理なく意思疎通ができるようになるに違いありません。

バリー・ブラム医学博士

Contents

本書の構成と使い方 ……………………………………………………… 8
音声 CD の活用法 ………………………………………………………… 10

PART 1 基礎編

Chapter 0 - 病院概要
1 院内組織 ……………………………………………………… 12
2 受診の手順 …………………………………………………… 14
3 院内順路案内 ………………………………………………… 16

Chapter 1 - 総合受付
1 初診患者 ……………………………………………………… 18
2 初診受付 ……………………………………………………… 20
3 再診受付 ……………………………………………………… 25
4 初診受付(一般診療所) ……………………………………… 26
5 診療科受付 …………………………………………………… 28

Chapter 2 - 問診
1 症状をたずねる ……………………………………………… 32
2 症状を詳しくたずねる ……………………………………… 36
3 日常の習慣をたずねる ……………………………………… 40
4 既往歴・家族歴をたずねる ………………………………… 44

Chapter 3 - 身体診察
1 視診・聴診・触診を行う …………………………………… 48
2 バイタルサインの評価を行う ……………………………… 52

Chapter 4 - 検査
1 検査を指示する ……………………………………………… 56
2 採血・尿検査をする ………………………………………… 60
3 さまざまな検査をする ……………………………………… 64

Chapter 5 - 診断・処置・処方
1 検査結果を伝える …………………………………………… 70
2 処方箋を出す ………………………………………………… 74
3 次の予約を入れる …………………………………………… 78

Chapter 6 - 手術・入院
　　　　1 必要性・注意事項を説明する ─── 82
　　　　2 麻酔について質問・説明する ─── 86

Chapter 7 - 会計
　　　　1 会計窓口 ─── 88

Chapter 8 - ER（救急治療室）
　　　　1 救急措置 ─── 92

PART 2　応用編

内科系

Chapter 1 - 神経内科
　　　　1 神経痛 ─── 98
　　　　2 頭痛 ─── 102

Chapter 2 - 消化器内科
　　　　1 潰瘍性大腸炎 ─── 106
　　　　2 胃潰瘍 ─── 110

Chapter 3 - 腎臓内科
　　　　1 腎臓病 ─── 114

Chapter 4 - 呼吸器内科
　　　　1 慢性閉塞性肺疾患 ─── 118
　　　　2 閉塞性睡眠時無呼吸 ─── 124

Chapter 5 - 循環器内科
　　　　1 心臓疾患 (1) ─── 128
　　　　2 心臓疾患 (2) ─── 132
　　　　3 高血圧症 ─── 136
　　　　4 動脈硬化 ─── 140

Chapter 6 - 血液内科
- 1 リンパ腫 —— 146
- 2 悪性貧血 —— 150

Chapter 7 - 糖尿病代謝内科
- 1 糖尿病 —— 154

Chapter 8 - 精神科
- 1 摂食障害 —— 158
- 2 うつ病 —— 162
- 3 双極性障害 —— 166

Chapter 9 - リウマチ科
- 1 関節リウマチ —— 170

外科系

Chapter 10 - 一般外科
- 1 虫垂炎 —— 174
- 2 胆石 —— 178
- 3 腰痛・背痛 —— 182

Chapter 11 - 整形外科
- 1 捻挫・骨折 —— 186
- 2 傷 —— 190
- 3 ヘルニア —— 194
- 4 手根管症候群 —— 198

Chapter 12 - 心臓血管外科
- 1 虚血性心疾患 —— 202

Chapter 13 - 脳神経外科
- 1 てんかん —— 206
- 2 脳卒中 —— 210
- 3 アルツハイマー病 —— 214

Chapter 14 - 乳腺外科
- 1 乳腺腫瘍 —— 218

その他

Chapter 15 – 小児科
1 ぜんそく・インフルエンザ ………… 222

Chapter 16 – 肛門科
1 痔核 ………… 226

Chapter 17 – 産婦人科
1 子宮筋腫 ………… 230
2 分娩 ………… 234

Chapter 18 – 泌尿器科
1 膀胱炎 ………… 238
2 前立腺肥大 ………… 242

Chapter 19 – 形成外科
1 顔面神経麻痺 ………… 246

Chapter 20 – 皮膚科
1 皮膚アレルギー ………… 250
2 できもの ………… 254
3 抜け毛 ………… 258

Chapter 21 – 眼科
1 ドライアイ ………… 262
2 白内障 ………… 266

Chapter 22 – 耳鼻咽喉科
1 めまい・耳鳴り ………… 270
2 メニエール病 ………… 274
3 鼻炎・副鼻腔炎 ………… 278
4 耳感染症 ………… 282

Chapter 23 – 歯科・口腔外科
1 歯根管 ………… 286

医療用語リスト ………… 291

本書の構成と使い方

本書は PART 1『基礎編』と PART 2『応用編』の 2 つのパートで構成されています。PART 1 で基本表現をマスターし、PART 2 では PART 1 で学習した基本フレーズをふまえて、各診療科に特化した専門性の高い診療会話を身につけていきます。

PART 1

患者さんが病院の門をくぐってから、診察を受け、会計を済ませるまでの流れに沿って、病院内で医師をはじめとする病院スタッフが外国人患者に応対する英語表現が掲載されています。

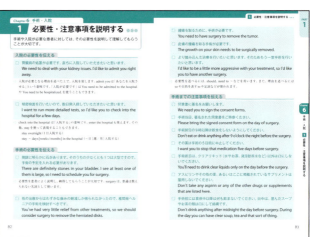

目的別に診療シーンで使えるフレーズ

日本語→英語で掲載されています。必要なフレーズを見つけたいときにも便利です。

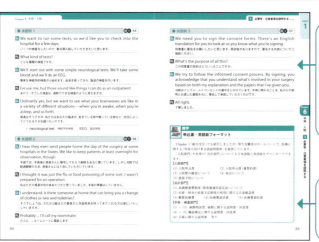

基本フレーズを使ったミニ会話例

実際の場面でどのように使うか、音声を聞きながら確認できます。

多様なコラム

医療の知識や表現の使い方を学べます。

本書の構成と使い方

PART 2

各診療科での会話例です。ここでは、南弘前病院という架空の病院の診療科で日常繰り広げられる会話で構成されています。

診察場面の会話例
実践に即した患者さんとのやり取りが身につけられます。会話はCDに吹き込まれていますので、繰り返し聞いて、ナチュラルなスピードに慣れてください。

訳
日英対訳になっています。

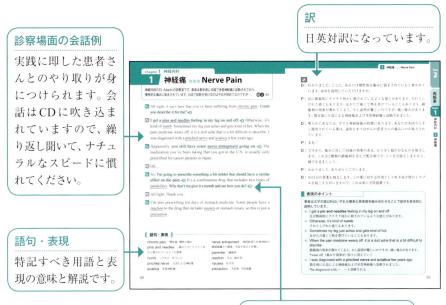

語句・表現
特記すべき用語と表現の意味と解説です。

❋はポイントとなる表現です。

❋は会話で使われている表現です。

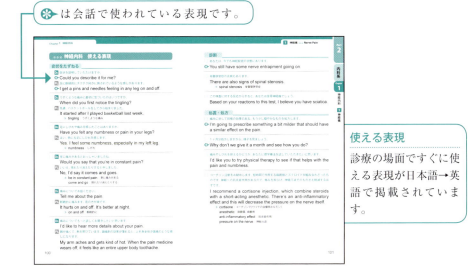

使える表現
診療の場面ですぐに使える表現が日本語→英語で掲載されています。

音声CDの活用法

CD 1にPART 1の会話例、CD 2にPART 2の会話が収録されています。会話ごとにトラックを分けて収録されていますので、必要なところから開始することができます。

● CD 1 CD 1 (PART 1) の活用法
CD 1には日本語での会話も収録されています。英語を聞いたあと、意味を確認することで、しっかりと基本表現を定着させることができます。

● CD 2 CD 2 (PART 2) の活用法
CD 2は診療科別のより専門性の高い会話が収録されています。実際の医療場面で使われるナチュラルスピードになっていますので、繰り返し聞くことで実践で役立つ診療英語を身につけることができます。

トラック一覧

CD 1

Chapter 0 …… 病院概要	Tr 01 〜 02
Chapter 1 …… 総合受付	Tr 03 〜 15
Chapter 2 …… 問診	Tr 16 〜 27
Chapter 3 …… 身体診察	Tr 28 〜 34
Chapter 4 …… 検査	Tr 35 〜 47
Chapter 5 …… 診断・処置・処方	Tr 48 〜 54
Chapter 6 …… 手術・入院	Tr 55 〜 59
Chapter 7 …… 会計	Tr 60 〜 62
Chapter 8 …… ER (救急治療室)	Tr 63 〜 69

CD 2

Chapter 1 …… 神経内科	Tr 01 〜 02
Chapter 2 …… 消化器内科	Tr 03 〜 04
Chapter 3 …… 腎臓内科	Tr 05
Chapter 4 …… 呼吸器内科	Tr 06 〜 07
Chapter 5 …… 循環器内科	Tr 08 〜 11
Chapter 6 …… 血液内科	Tr 12 〜 13
Chapter 7 …… 糖尿病代謝内科	Tr 14
Chapter 8 …… 精神科	Tr 15 〜 17
Chapter 9 …… リウマチ科	Tr 18
Chapter 10 …… 一般外科	Tr 19 〜 21
Chapter 11 …… 整形外科	Tr 22 〜 25
Chapter 12 …… 心臓血管外科	Tr 26
Chapter 13 …… 脳神経外科	Tr 27 〜 29
Chapter 14 …… 乳腺外科	Tr 30
Chapter 15 …… 小児科	Tr 31
Chapter 16 …… 肛門科	Tr 32
Chapter 17 …… 産婦人科	Tr 33 〜 34
Chapter 18 …… 泌尿器科	Tr 35 〜 36
Chapter 19 …… 形成外科	Tr 37
Chapter 20 …… 皮膚科	Tr 38 〜 40
Chapter 21 …… 眼科	Tr 41 〜 42
Chapter 22 …… 耳鼻咽喉科	Tr 43 〜 46
Chapter 23 …… 歯科・口腔外科	Tr 47

PART 1 基礎編

『南弘前総合病院』を舞台に、
患者が病院のエントランスをくぐり、
検査や診断などの必要な処置を受けて
会計を済ませるまでの流れに沿って構成されています。
挨拶や患者の症状を聞くなど、
すべての病院関係者が使える基本表現を
まず身につけましょう。

Chapter 0 - 病院概要

1 院内組織

南弘前総合病院の診療科を紹介します。院長・副院長の下に、病院には次のような診療科があります。

● 南弘前総合病院　Minami Hirosaki General Hospital

院長　　橋本太郎　　　Taro Hashimoto, Director General
副院長　秋山玲奈　　　Reina Akiyama, Assistant Director

診療科	Hospital Departments
神経内科	Neurology
消化器内科	Gastroenterology
腎臓内科	Nephrology
呼吸器内科	Respiratory Medicine
循環器内科	Cardiovascular Medicine
血液内科	Hematology
糖尿病代謝内科	Endocrinology and Metabolism
精神科	Psychiatry
小児科	Pediatrics
リウマチ科	Rheumatology
肛門科	Proctology
泌尿器科	Urology
産婦人科	Obstetrics and Gynecology
一般外科	General Surgery
整形外科	Orthopedic Surgery
心臓血管外科	Cardiovascular Surgery
脳神経外科	Neurosurgery
形成外科	Plastic Surgery
乳腺外科	Breast Surgery
皮膚科	Dermatology
眼科	Ophthalmology
耳鼻咽喉科	Otorhinolaryngology
歯科・口腔外科	Dentistry and Oral Surgery
救急外来	Emergency Room: ER

診察設備　Laboratory & Other facilities

診察設備	Laboratory and Other facilities
検査部門	Laboratory
リハビリテーション	Rehabilitation
放射線	Radiology
集中治療室(ICU)	Intensive Care Unit (ICU)
手術室	Operating Room
健康診断	Health Examinations

薬剤部　Pharmacy

看護部　Nursing Department

雑学
診療科の名前（語幹について）

医学用語は、ギリシャ語やラテン語を語源に持ちます。診療科の名前の多くは学問名が用いられているため、「～学・～術」を意味する「-ology」や「-ics」がついたものが多く見られます。

神経内科	Neur+ology
腎臓内科	Nephr+ology
血液内科	Hemat+ology
糖尿病代謝内科	Endocrin+ology
小児科	Pediat+rics
肛門科	Proct+ology
リウマチ科	Rheumat+ology
整形外科	Orthop(a)ed+ics
産婦人科	Obstetr+ics and Gynec+ology
泌尿器科	Ur+ology
皮膚科	Dermat+ology
眼科	Ophthalm+ology
耳鼻咽喉科	Otorhinolaryng+ology

Chapter 0 — 病院概要

2　受診の手順

南弘前病院では、病院を訪れた患者は、以下の手順で診察を受けます。救急時以外は、全科予約診療となっています。Chapter 1以降では、この受診の手順に沿って、それぞれの場面で必要な会話を紹介します。

● 受診の手順　Flow Chart

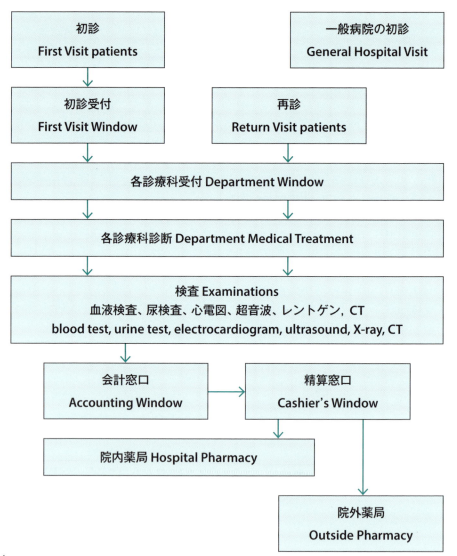

> **雑学**
> ### 外国人患者受け入れの3つの課題「言語対応」「未収金」「安全管理」
>
> 　国際化社会を迎えた今日、日本に往来、居住する外国人の増加によって、医療機関を受診する外国人も増加したことから、医療機関においては外国人患者への対応や受け入れ体制が求められるようになりました。こうしたことから、厚生労働省は、国際的に高い評価を得ている日本の医療サービスを外国人が安心・安全に受けることのできる体制作りのため、支援事業として、「外国人患者受入れ医療機関認証制度（JAIP: Japan Medical Service Accreditation for International Patients）」を立ち上げています。
> 　当認証制度の認証機関である日本医療教育財団は、2012年10月に行われたセミナーで、病院が外国人患者を受け入れる上で、「言語対応」「未収金」「安全管理」の3つの課題を指摘しています。
> 　課題のひとつ、「言語対応」では以下の点が例示されました。
>
> 　「日本語での対応が難しい外国人が来院した場合、担当者が明確になっていないために現場が混乱し、兼務で対応する職員の本来業務が圧迫される。通訳者を付ける場合にも、現場の認識不足、現場スタッフが外国人の話す言葉がまったくわからないため、通訳の精度が担保できない。」
> 　「解決策としては、専任の担当者を置く、電話通訳を活用する、自治体と連携、低コストで通訳を付けるといったことが考えられる。また、医療機関・通訳者・外国人患者の3者で、通訳を介する診療のリスクを書面で共有したり、外国人患者に通訳サービスの満足度調査を行うことも必要だと考えられる。」

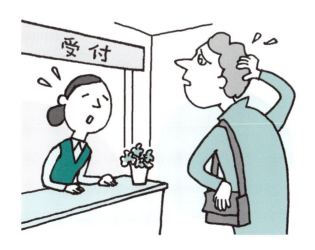

Chapter 0 - 病院概要

3　院内順路案内

大病院では、訪れた患者が迷うことがよくあります。Chapter 1に入る前に、院内案内図をもとに順路案内の表現を紹介します。

● 南弘前病院1階案内図

　救急外来の患者以外は、初診でも再診でも、まずは1階の受付を通ることになります。順路をたずねる患者は正面玄関を背に受付の前に立っています。

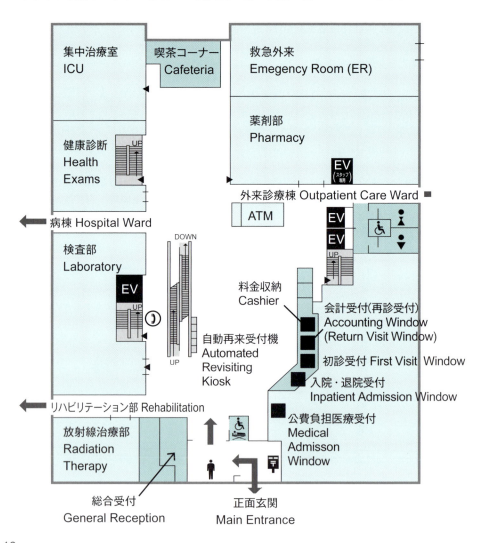

順路を案内する

- 右［左］に曲がってください／右［左］です。
  Turn right [left]. / It's on the right [left].

- 〜の前です／〜の後ろです。
  It's in front of 〜 / It's behind 〜

- 〜の角を曲がったところです。
  It's around the corner 〜

- このホールの突き当たりにあります。
  It's at the end of this hall.

- エレベーターで3階に上がってください。
  Take the elevator up to the 3rd floor.

● 会話例 1

F.P. Can you tell me how to get to the pharmacy?
薬剤部への行き方を教えてくださいますか。

Re. Do you see the ATM over there? The pharmacy is behind the ATM.
あそこのATMが見えますか。薬剤部はATMの後ろです。

● 会話例 2

F.P. Where do I go to have a health exam?
健康診断を受けるにはどこへ行けばいいですか。

Re. Go straight along this hall and past the escalator. You'll see the health exam room on your left.
このホールをまっすぐ進み、エスカレーターを通り過ぎてください。健康診断室は左側です。

Chapter 1 - 総合受付

1 初診患者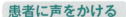

初診、再診、面会…、受付に立ち寄る人の目的はさまざまです。ここでは、総合病院を初診で訪れた患者への対応を紹介します。

患者に声をかける

☐ どうなさいましたか。
　May I help you?

⇨ 病院の受付に立ち寄る人、全般に対して使います。まずMay I help you? とこちらから声をかけて、話のきっかけを作ります。

☐ 当院へいらしたのは初めてですか。
　Is this your first visit to our hospital?

⇨ 総合病院の入口を入ると、日本人でも勝手がわからないものです。外来では、初診（first visit）と再診（return visit）で手続きが違うので、初診と思われるような患者には、Is this your first visit 〜? と声をかけます。また、再診であっても、多くの病院で、前回診察を受けてから数ヶ月経つと、初診扱いになります。

☐ 当院に前回来たときから３ヶ月経っていたら、もう一度初診の手続きが必要です。
　If you have not been back to the hospital in three months, you need to repeat the first visit procedure.

総合病院で初診を受け付ける条件を確認する

☐ 紹介状はお持ちですか。
　Did you bring a letter of introduction?

☐ 医師の紹介状をお持ちですか。
　Do you have a referral from another doctor?

☐ 予約はなさっていますか。
　Do you have an appointment?

⇨ 予約にはappointmentを使います。reservationを用いるとレストランなどの予約のように聞こえてしまいます。

▶ letter of introduction, medical referral certificate：紹介状

1 初診患者

- ☐ 本院での治療を希望される場合には、前任の医師の紹介状（診療情報提供書）をご提示いただく必要があります。
  In order to be treated at this hospital, you need to submit a referral from your previous doctor that includes treatment information.

- ☐ 本院では、小児科と一般外科以外は、紹介状がないと受診できません。
  At this hospital, with the exception of the Pediatrics and General Surgery departments, you can't consult a doctor without the letter of introduction.

- ☐ 初診料として特別に4320円が必要です。この費用は、健康保険では補填されません。
  A special fee of 4,320 yen will be charged for your first consultation. This fee is not covered by your national health insurance plan.

- ☐ 救急の場合を除いて、どの診療科で診察を受ける場合でも予約が必要です。事前に予約をお願いします。
  Except for emergency cases, all consultations in all departments are conducted by appointment. Please make an appointment in advance.

● 会話例 1　　CD 1 -03

Re. May I help you? Is this your first visit to our hospital?
どうなさいましたか。当院へいらしたのは初めてですか。

Pt. Yes.
はい。

Re. Did you bring a letter of introduction?
紹介状はお持ちですか。

Pt. Yes, here it is.
はい、ここに。

Re. You need to go to the initial appointment registration area first. It's over there, at Window No.1.
まず初診受付へ行ってください。初診受付は、あそこの1番窓口です。

Chapter 1 - 総合受付

2 初診受付 •••

初めて当病院を訪れた患者は、初診の受付で診察申込書の記入、健康保険証の提示など必要な手続きを行います。

診察申込書 (Registration Form)

☐ 外来の診察申込書を記入していただけますか。
　Could you fill out the outpatient registration form for us?

☐ この申込書を記入していただけますか。
　Would you mind filling out this form?

⇨ 初診の患者には、最初に「診察申込書」(registration form) に記入してもらいます。Could [Would] you ～? を使って丁寧に対応しましょう。Would you mind ～ing? を使えば、もっと丁寧な表現になります。Please fill out the registration form for outpatients. と言うこともできます。申込書のように「空欄に何かを記入する」場合には、fill out を使います。もしとっさに出てこなければ、Please fill this out. を丁寧な調子で言えばよいでしょう。

健康保険証 (Health Insurance Card)

☐ 日本の健康保険証をお持ちですか。
　・Do you have a Japanese health insurance card?
　・Do you have Japanese insurance?

⇨ 診察申込書に名前や住所などを記入してもらったら、「健康保険証 (health insurance card)」を提出してもらいます。医師の紹介状もこのときに提出してもらいます。

☐ 健康保険証を提出してください。保険証を提出なさらない場合には、医療費を全額お支払いいただくことになります。
　Please present your health insurance card. We'll need to ask you to pay the full amount of the medical fees if an insurance card is not presented.

☐ あなたは日本に旅行中のようですね。旅行保険に加入していますか。
　You seem to be a visitor to Japan. Do you have travel insurance?

診察券（Hospital ID card）

□ 診察券を持って、指定された診療科受付に行ってください。
　Please take your hospital ID to the designated department.

⇨ 一通りの書類を受付に提出すると、患者の診察券（hospital ID）が用意されます。用意されている間に、今度は「問診票（medical questionnaire）」を記入してもらいます。

● 会話例1

Re. Good morning. May I have your name, please?
こんにちは。お名前を教えていただけますか。

Pt. It's Nancy Baxter.
ナンシー・バクスターです。

Re. Do you have Japanese health insurance?
日本の健康保険証をお持ちですか。

Pt. Yes. Here you go.
はい。これです。

● 会話例2

Re. Could you fill out the outpatient registration form?
外来用の診察申込書に記入していただけますか。

Pt. I can't read Japanese.
日本語が読めないのですが。

Re. There's an English sample over at the counter. You can refer to that. If there's anything that you don't understand, please let us know.
あちらのカウンターに英語のサンプルがあります。それを参考にしてください。わからないことがあったら、教えてください。

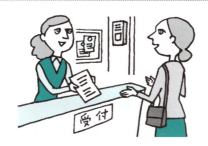

会話例 3

Re. We need your registration form, your insurance card and a letter of introduction.
診断申込書、健康保険証、それから紹介状を提出してください。

Pt. Here are my documents.
はい、これです。

Re. Thank you. Please have a seat while we prepare your hospital ID card.
ありがとうございます。診察券を用意する間、おかけになってお待ちください。

Pt. Sure.
わかりました。

会話例 4

Re. While you're waiting, would you fill out this medical history questionnaire? We have an English version.
お待ちになっている間に、この問診票を記入してくださいますか。英語版があります。

Pt. Sure.
はい。

Re. Ms. Baxter, here's your hospital ID card. You need to bring this ID card with you every time you visit our hospital.
バクスターさん、こちらが診察券です。当院にいらっしゃる時にはいつもこの診察券を持ってきてください。

Pt. What do I do next?
次に何をすればよいですか。

Re. Please take the hospital ID and this printout to the designated department.
診察券とこのプリントアウトを持って、指定された診療科に行ってください。

▶ hospital ID：診察券　　medical questionnaire：問診票

● 診察申込書（Registration Form）

　外国人向けの書式を用意していない病院も多いでしょう。厚生労働省はホームページで、医療に関する「外国人向け多言語説明資料」を提供しており、診察申込書、各科の問診票、発生する支払いに関する資料などをダウンロードすることができます。
http://www.mhlw.go.jp/stf/seisakunitsuite/bunya/0000056789.html

診療申込書（日本語版）

```
患者氏名：
患者ID：                                                          日本語 / 日本語

                          診療申込書

氏名                                    性別              □男  □女
生年月日      年    月    日            年齢                      歳
住所又は日本での滞在先
〒

本国の住所（短期滞在者のみ）


電話（自宅）                    電話（携帯）
国籍                            通訳の希望        □必要    □必要でない
母国語                          職業
母国語以外に                    宗教上の理由により
対応可能な言語                  特別に配慮が必要な事項

緊急連絡先
氏名                                    患者との関係
住所
電話（自宅）                    電話（携帯）

●日本での滞在状況を教えて下さい。
    □居住  □短期滞在（□ビジネス  □旅行）  □留学生  □その他（        ）
●当院をお選びいただいた理由を教えてください。

●当院のご受診は初めてですか。       □はい    □いいえ
●紹介状はありますか。               □あり    □なし
●予約はしていますか。               □あり    □なし
保険の種類
    □日本の保険    （□公的保険    □プライベート保険）
    □海外の保険    （保険会社名：                          ）
              ※保険証や関連書類をお持ちの場合はご提示ください。
    □保険に加入していない
希望される診療科
  □整形外科  □心療内科  □耳鼻科  □皮膚科  □内科  □外科  □歯科  □眼科  □脳神経外科
  □小児科  □産婦人科  □呼吸器科  □呼吸器外科  □循環器科  □心臓血管外科  □消化器科
  □腎臓内科  □泌尿器科  □神経内科

※患者様の個人情報については、院内の規定に基づき対応させていただきます。

                                        診療申込書：2014年3月初版
```

Chapter 1 - 総合受付

診療申込書（英語版）

患者氏名 ：
患者ID ：

English/英語

PATIENT REGISTRATION FORM

Name		Sex	☐Male ☐Female
Date of birth (YYYY/MM/DD)	/ /	Age	years old

Address or accommodation in Japan

Address in home country (for short-term visitors only)

Phone No. (Home)		Phone No. (Mobile)		
Nationality		Interpreter request	☐Yes	☐No
Native language		Occupation		
Other languages spoken		Special requirements for religious reasons		

Emergency contact details

Name		Relationship	
Address			
Phone No. (Home)		Phone No. (Mobile)	

● Immigration status in Japan
　☐Resident　☐Short-term stay (☐Business　☐Vacation)　☐Student　☐Other (　　　　)
● Reasons for choosing this hospital/clinic

● Is this your first visit to this hospital/clinic?　☐Yes　☐No
● Do you have a referral letter?　☐Yes　☐No
● Do you have an appointment?　☐Yes　☐No

Type of health insurance

　☐Japanese health insurance　(☐public　☐private)
　☐Overseas health insurance (name of insurance company:　　　　　　　　　　)
　　Please present your insurance certificate or related documents if available.
　☐Uninsured

Medical departments you would like to visit

☐Orthopedics　☐Psychosomatic Medicine　☐Otorhinolaryngology　☐Dermatology　☐Internal Medicine
☐Surgery　☐Dentistry　☐Ophthalmology　☐Neurosurgery　☐Pediatrics　☐Obstetrics and Gynecology
☐Respiratory Medicine　☐Thoracic Surgery　☐Cardiology　☐Cardiovascular Surgery　☐Gastroenterology
☐Nephrology　☐Urology　☐Neurology

*Your personal information will be handled in accordance with the regulations of the institution.

診療申込書 ： 2014年3月初版

Chapter 1 - 総合受付

3　再診受付

再診（return visit）の外来患者は、すでに診察券を持っているので、初診（first visit）よりも手続きが簡略化されます。

- ☐ 受付機に診察券を入れてください。
  Please insert your hospital ID card into the machine.

- ☐ ここにあるボックスに診察券を入れてください。
  Please put your hospital ID in the box here.

⇨ 総合病院では、コンピュータ管理されているところも多く、自動受付機に診察券を入れればそれで受付は終了です。もちろん診察券を所定のボックスに入れる病院も多くあります。

- ☐ 何か身分証明書を見せていただけますか。
  Can I see some ID?

- ☐ 身分証明書（パスポート、在留カード、免許証）を見せていただけますか。
  May I see your (passport, resident card, driver's license)?

- ☐ 緊急の場合に連絡が取れる電話番号を教えていただけますか。
  May I have a number we can contact in case of emergency?

● 会話例 1　

Pt. I'd like to see Dr. Suzuki in General Surgery.
一般外科の鈴木先生の診察を受けたいのですが。

Re. Please insert your hospital ID card into the machine; take the check-in slip and proceed to the designated department.
診察券を自動受付機に差し込み、受付票を取ったら、指定された診療科に進んでください。

Chapter 1 - 総合受付

4 初診受付（一般診療所）

ここまで規模の大きな総合病院での初診・再診の受付手順を見てきましたが、最後に規模の小さな一般の診療クリニックの受付についても触れておきましょう。

☐ （初診の）登録受付を済ませてください。
Please check in with registration.

⇒ 規模の大きな病院とは異なり、多くのクリニックの受付は1カ所だけです。初診でも再診でも、来院した患者は、受付で診察に必要な手続きをまとめて済ませます。
　こうした診療クリニックの受付では、英語版の「診察申込書（registration form）」「問診票（medical questionnaire）」を用意しておき、訪れた患者に記入してもらうやり方が効率がよいと思われます。

● 会話例 1

Re. Good morning. May I help you?
おはようございます。どうなさいましたか。

Pt. I seem to have caught a cold. I can't stop coughing.
風邪を引いたようです。咳が止まりません。

Re. Please put on this mask. It's a precaution against infection. Do you have Japanese health insurance?
このマスクをしてください。感染予防のためです。日本の健康保険証はお持ちですか。

Pt. Actually I don't. I'm here on business.
実は持っていません。出張で来ているのです。

Re. I see. You'll have to pay the entire cost of treatment yourself. Will that be all right?
なるほど。全額自費診療になりますが、よろしいですか。

Pt. I have travel insurance. I'll just need to get a medical certificate and a receipt from you.
私は旅行保険に入っています。診断書と領収書をいただければ結構です。

Re. Sure. We'll give those to you at the cashier after you've seen the doctor.
承知しました。診察後に会計でお渡しします。

▶ precaution against infection：感染予防　　cost of treatment：治療費
　travel insurance：旅行保険　　medical certificate：診断書

● 会話例 2

Re. Good morning. May I help you?
おはようございます。どうなさいましたか。

Pt. Yes. I've had a stomachache since last night, so I'd like to see a doctor.
はい。昨晩からお腹が痛くて、先生の診断を受けたいのですが。

Re. Is this your first visit to this hospital?
当院へいらしたのは初めてですか。

Pt. Yes. I just moved here from Hong Kong last month.
はい。先月香港からこちらに引っ越してきたところです。

Re. Do you have Japanese health insurance?
日本の健康保険証はお持ちですか。

Pt. Yes, here's my card.
はい、これです。

Re. You'll need to check in with registration. Please fill out this form over there and bring it with you.
初診の登録を済ませてください。あちらでこの用紙を記入したら、お持ちください。

Pt. I see.
わかりました。

Re. Once you've completed the registration, we'll send you to the department of the doctor you wish to see.
登録が完了したら、診察を希望なさっている診療科の先生のところにご案内します。

Chapter 1 - 総合受付

5　診療科受付

初診・再診の受付を済ませ、目的の診療科受付にやってきた患者への対応表現を紹介します。診療科での待ち時間の長さに適切な対応をとる必要があります。

診察券の提示を促す

- [ ] カウンターに診察券を提出してください。受付番号をお渡しします。
  Please present your hospital ID card at the counter. You'll get a check-in number.

⇨ 診察券（IDカード）で管理・運営する病院がほとんどですから、外来受付ではまず患者に診察券の提出を促します。

- [ ] 診察券をこのボックスに入れてください。
  Please put your hospital ID card in this box.

- [ ] 診察券をこの受付機に挿入してください。
  Please insert your hospital ID card into this machine.

受付手順を説明する

- [ ] お名前を呼ばれるまで、ここでお待ちください。
  Please wait here until you are called.

- [ ] お名前を呼ばれたら5番の部屋にお入りください。
  When you are called, please go to Room 5.

- [ ] 受付番号を呼ばれたら、5番の部屋にお入りください。
  When your check-in number is called, please go to Room 5.

- [ ] 待っている間に、気分が悪くなったら申し出てください。
  Please tell us if you feel sick while you're waiting.

- [ ] 気分がさらに悪化し出したら申し出てください。
  If you start to feel worse, please let us know.

5 診療科受付

待ち時間を説明する

- □ もう少しお待ちください。
  Please wait just a little longer.

- □ 受付順に患者さんを診察するようにしています。
  We try to see patients in the order of check-in.

- □ 予期せぬ事情で診療が遅れることがありますのでご理解ください。
  Please understand that consultations can be delayed due to a variety of unforeseen circumstances.

⇨ 待ち時間が長くなって、患者がいらいらするといった状況では、不安を取り除くべく、できるだけ穏やかな口調で言う必要があります。

順番が来たことを知らせる

- □ 受付番号36番の患者様、5番の診察室にお入りください。
  Check-in number 36, please go to Room 5.

⇨ 外国人患者の場合、名前を正確に発音することが困難な場合があります。受付番号で診察の順番が来たことを知らせる方が確実です。

- □ アリス・スミス様、順番がきました。どうぞお入りください。
  Ms. Alice Smith, the doctor can see you now. Please go in.

⇨ 番号が表示されても、番号が呼ばれても、気が付かない患者さんもおられます。そうしたときにこのように声掛けします。

- □ まだ順番ではありません。
  I'm afraid it's not your turn yet.

⇨ I'm afraidを前につけると少し柔らかい表現になります。

名前が読みにくい場合

- □ お名前[名字]はどう発音しますか。
  How do you pronounce your first [last] name?

- □ お名前を正しく言えていますか。
  Am I saying it right?

⇨ Ms. Alice Smithといった具合に、患者さんの名前をフルネームではっきり呼ぶこ

29

とは、本人かどうかを確認する意味でも大切です。一度確認したら、次からは Ms. Smith のように姓で呼べばよいでしょう。

　また、外国人の名前はどう発音したらよいのかわからない場合もあります。名前の読み方は、受付時や順番待ちの間に、本人に確認しておくとよいでしょう。

● 会話例 1

Pt. Excuse me. This is my first visit to this department.
すみません。この診療科に初診で来たのですが。

N Please insert your hospital ID card into this machine. You'll get a print-out with your check-in number.
この受付機に診察券を入れてください。受付番号の書かれたプリントアウトが出てきます。

Pt. Oh, all right.
ああ、わかりました。

N Check-in numbers will be displayed on a screen in the waiting room. Watching the display will probably help you estimate the time remaining until your consultation.
受付番号が待合室の掲示板に表示されます。掲示板を見ていれば、診察までの大まかな待ち時間を予測できるでしょう。

● 会話例 2

N How are you feeling at the moment?
今、ご気分はいかがですか。

Pt. I don't feel so bad right now, but I'd like to see the doctor as soon as possible.
今のところそれほど悪くはないですが、なるべく早く先生に診てもらいたいと思います。

N We try to see patients in the order of check-in, but please let us know if you start to feel sick while you're waiting.
私どもは受付順に患者さんを診察するようにしていますが、待っている間に、気分が悪くなったら申し出てください。

Pt. OK.
わかりました。

会話例 3

N Would you mind having a seat? The doctor will be with you shortly.
おかけになっていただけますか。まもなく先生が診察いたします。

Pt. OK. Thanks.
わかりました。ありがとう。

会話例 4

Pt. Listen, I've been waiting here for more than an hour. How much longer will I need to wait for my turn?
すみません、1時間以上待っているのです。私の順番まであとどのくらい待たなければならないでしょうか。

N Let me go find out.
確認してまいります。

N We can probably call you in 30 minutes.
30分ほどでお呼びできると思います。

Pt. Uh... 30 more minutes?
えっ、あと30分もですか。

N Please understand that consultations can be delayed due to a variety of unforeseen circumstances.
予期せぬ事情で診療が遅れることがありますのでご理解ください。

会話例 5

N Mr. Giovanni Tiepolo, the doctor can see you now. Please go to Room 5.
ジョバンニ・ティエポロ様、順番がきました。5番の部屋にお入りください。

Dr. Good morning, Mr. Tiepolo. Please come in. I'm Dr. Shimizu.
おはようございます、ティエポロさん。お入りください。医師の清水です。

Pt. Good morning.
おはようございます。

Chapter 2 - 問診

1 症状をたずねる

問診の基本は症状を正確に聞き出すことです。最初に患者の来院の目的をたずねます。

来院の目的をたずねる

☐ どうなさいましたか。
- What's the problem [trouble]?
- What seems to be the problem [trouble]?

⇨ seems to ~ を使うことで What's the problem [trouble]? よりも柔らかい印象を与えることができます。

☐ 今日はどうなさったのですか。
- What brings you here today?
- What brings you in today?

⇨ 直訳すると「何があなたをここへ連れてきたのですか」で、受診の目的をたずねます。間接的な表現が患者さんに安心感を与えます。

具体的な症状を聞く

☐ 何が問題か具体的に話していただけますか。
Could you tell me what exactly is the problem?

⇨ What exactly is the problem? だと直接的すぎるので、Could you tell me をつけるとよいでしょう。

☐ 痛みについて話してください。
Can you describe the pain for me?

⇨ 症状を詳しく聞くときには、describe を使います。

☐ 何があったか話してください。
Tell me about what happened?

☐ どこが痛みますか。
Where does it hurt?

⇨ 外傷など急いで処置をする必要がある場合に使います。

●●● 患者が症状を訴える表現

寒気 ………	ぞくぞくします。 **I have the chills.** 寒気がひどいのです。 **I feel very cold.**
熱 …………	微熱［高熱］があります。 **I have a slight [high] fever.** 熱が38.5℃あります。 **My temperature is thirty-eight point five degrees.**
喉の痛み ……	喉が痛みます。 **I have a sore throat.**
鼻づまり ……	鼻がつまっています。 **My nose is stuffed up.**
鼻水 ………	鼻水が出ます。 **I have a runny nose.**
咳 …………	咳が出ます。　＊咳は何回出ても、have a cough と単数形です。 **I have a cough.**
食欲不振 ……	ここ1ヶ月ほど、食欲がありません。 **My appetite has been poor for the past month.** **I haven't been able to eat much for the past month.**
下痢 ………	下痢をしています。 **I have diarrhea.**
体重が減る …	ここ1ヶ月で2キロ痩せました。 **I've lost 2 kg in the last month.**
吐き気 ……	胃がむかむかして、吐き気がします。 **I have an upset stomach and nausea.**
むくみ ……	顔が少しむくんでいます。 **My face has been a little puffy.** 足がむくみます。 **My legs are swollen.**
かゆみ ……	目がかゆいです。 **My eyes are itchy.** かゆみはときどき耐えられないことがあります。 **The itching is sometimes quite unbearable.**

Chapter 2 - 問診

冷え	………	腰から足にかけて冷えます。
		My lower back and legs have been feeling cold.
疲れ	………	最近疲れがひどいです。
		I feel very tired these days.
しこり	………	首のところにしこりを感じました。
		I felt a lump in my neck.
発疹	………	発疹があります。
		I have a rash.
息切れ	………	息切れがします。
		I'm having shortness of breath.
転落	………	階段から落ちました。
		I fell down the stairs.
捻挫	………	足首［手首］を捻挫しました。
		I twisted my ankle [wrist].
		I sprained my ankle [wrist].
骨折	………	腕を折りました。
		I broke my arm.
		My arm is broken.

● 会話例 1　　　　　　　　　　　　　　　CD ①-16

Dr. Good morning. What seems to be the trouble?
おはようございます。どうなさいましたか。

Pt. My neck is killing me.
首がずっと痛くてたまりません。

▶ (be) killing me：耐えられない、死にそうだ

● 会話例 2　　　　　　　　　　　　　　　CD ①-17

Dr. Could you describe your problem, please?
症状を説明していただけますか。

Pt. I have an upset stomach and nausea.
胃がむかむかして吐き気がします。

会話例 3

Dr. Can you describe the pain for me?
痛みについて話していただけますか。

Pt. I have this ache in my right knee.
右膝にこの痛みがあります。

Pain from Head to Toe
痛みを表す用語（頭頂からつま先まで）

1. headache　　頭痛
2. earache　　耳痛
3. sinus pain　　副鼻腔の痛み
4. toothache　　歯痛
5. stiff neck　　首の痛み
    * 日本では「肩凝り」と言いますが、アメリカ人はむしろ首の方を強調します。

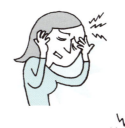

6. chest pains　　胸の痛み
7. heartburn [indigestion]　　胸やけ [消化不良]
8. stomachache　　胃痛
9. backache　　背中の痛み、腰痛
10. pain in the side　　脇腹の痛み
11. muscle aches　　筋肉痛

    * -ache の表記について
    古いゲルマン言語の名残で、一般的な体の部位に関する痛みの場合は、toothache や headache のように、1語で表記されます。しかし他の体の部位の痛みの場合は、muscle aches のように2語で表記されます。

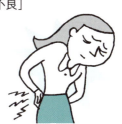

Chapter 2 - 問診

2 症状を詳しくたずねる

さらに詳しい症状を聞き出すための表現を見ていきます。症状の始まった時期、どのような痛みなのか、経過などを明らかにする質問をしていきます。

症状の始まった時期をたずねる

- □ いつ最初に痛みに気づきましたか。
  When did you first notice the pain?
- □ いつけがをしましたか。
  When did you injure yourself?

⇨ when を使って痛みや症状の開始時期をたずねます。これに対して患者は yesterday, two hours ago などで答えます。

継続期間をたずねる

- □ この問題ははどれくらい続いていますか。
  How long have you had this trouble [problem]?
- □ 症状はどれくらい続いていますか。
  How long have you had these symptoms?
- □ 具合が悪いのはどれくらい続いていますか。
  How long have you been feeling sick?
- □ 何時間、吐き気が続いていますか。
  How many hours has the nausea been going on?

⇨ 症状の継続期間をたずねる場合は、How long ～? / How many days [hours] ～? と現在完了を使います。患者は about two days, about three hours などと、期間で答えます。

- □ 痛みはどれくらい続いていますか。
  ・How long does the pain last?
  ・What's the duration of your headache?

⇨ last は「続く」という意味の動詞で、主語（症状）を変えて、How long does the headache last? などと使うことができます。

症状のある場所をたずねる

- ☐ どこが痛みますか。
  Where do you feel the pain?

- ☐ 具体的にどこにその発疹がありますか。
  Where exactly is the eruption?

⇨ Where で痛みや症状の場所をたずねます。

▶ eruption：発疹

状況や原因をたずねる

- ☐ どうやってけがをされましたか。
  How did you injure [hurt] yourself?

⇨ けがをした状況をたずねます。injure [hurt] は「〜を傷つける」という他動詞なので、「けがをする」というときはyourselfが必要です。具体的に部位を言う場合はHow did you injure your leg? と言います。

- ☐ 痛みの原因に心あたりはありますか。
  What do you think brought the pain on?

⇨ 痛みの原因が明確でない場合は do you think を使ってたずねます。

状況の起きる時期をたずねる

- ☐ 通常、いつ頭痛を感じますか。
  When do you usually get a headache?

- ☐ 1日のうちで痛みの変化はありますか。
  Does the pain change throughout the day?

⇨ 痛む時間帯や変化についてたずねる表現です。

痛みの程度をたずねる

- ☐ 痛みはどれくらいひどいですか。
  How severe is the pain?

- ☐ 痛みの程度はどれくらいですか。
  How bad is your pain?

⇨ 痛みの程度についてたずねる表現です。

Chapter **2** - 問診

> ☐ どんな種類の痛みですか。
> What kind of pain is it?

> ☐ どのような痛みですか。
> What is the pain like?

⇨ What kind of ~? / What ~ like? でどんな痛みかをたずねることができます。

> ☐ 激しい痛みですか、鈍い痛みですか。
> Is it a sharp pain or dull pain?

⇨ 痛みの表現には英語でも sharp pain（激しい、鋭い痛み）、dull pain（鈍い痛み）など決まった言い方があります。医師から提示すると患者は答えやすくなるので、覚えておくと役に立ちます。

● 会話例 1　　　　　　　　　　　　　　　　　　　　CD ①-19

Dr. How bad is your pain?
痛みの程度はどのくらいですか。

Pt. It's really bad. I think it keeps getting worse.
とてもひどいんです。だんだんと悪くなっているように思います。

Dr. What kind of pain is it?
どんな種類の痛みですか。

Pt. It's a throbbing pain.
ずきずきする痛みです。

● 会話例 2　　　　　　　　　　　　　　　　　　　　CD ①-20

Dr. How did it start?
その症状は、どのようにして始まりましたか。

Pt. My back was itchy and my mom saw I was broken out there.
背中にかゆみを覚え、母がそこに発疹を見つけたのです。

Dr. Where exactly is the eruption?
具体的にどこにその発疹がありますか。

Pt. It's here. (showing a spot on the back)
ここです。（背中を見せる）

2 症状を詳しくたずねる

● 会話例 3　　　CD 1 -21

Dr. Could you describe your pain for me?
痛みについて話していただけますか。

Pt. I have this tingling in my foot.
足にうずくような痛みがあります。

Dr. When did you first notice it?
その痛みに最初に気づいたのはいつですか。

Pt. It started after I played basketball last week.
先週、バスケットボールをしてから始まりました。

Dr. Let me take a look.
診せてください。

I feel 〜., I have 〜 pain.
具体的な痛みを表す言い方

＊印の語は後ろに pain をつけては使いません。

刺すような痛み	stabbing pain
うずくような痛み	*tingling; *feels like pins and needles
ずきずきする痛み	throbbing pain
刺し込む痛み	piercing pain
激しい痛み	sharp pain
鈍い痛み	dull pain
しつこい痛み	nagging pain
急性の痛み	acute pain
しびれて感覚がない	*numbness, *numb

Chapter 2 - 問診

3　日常の習慣をたずねる

患者の日常の生活習慣の把握は、適切な診断を下すために大切です。家庭、学校、仕事、嗜好などをたずねていきますが、患者が話しやすい雰囲気作りを心がけるようにします。

☐ 職業を伺ってもよろしいでしょうか。
　May I ask what your occupation is?

☐ ご結婚されているか伺ってもよろしいでしょうか。
　May I ask if you are married?

⇨ 英語圏では履歴書に年齢や家族状況は書かないのが慣例ですから、社会歴 (social history) をたずねる場合にも配慮が必要です。May I ask what 〜? / May I ask if 〜? などを使って丁寧に聞きます。

☐ 何か薬を服用していますか。
　・**Are you taking any medication?**
　・**Do you take any medication?**

⇨ 「薬」は medication や medicine を使います。drug は薬物とまぎらわしい場合には使い方に留意が必要です。ただし、患者と直接関係がない場合には、drug を使っても問題ありません。
　例) This drug has been tested for five years, so I feel comfortable recommending it to you.（この薬は5年間の治験を受けてきましたから、あなたに気兼ねなくおすすめできます）

☐ それをなさらないのは何か特別な理由がありますか。
　Is there any particular reason why not?

⇨ 患者の日常の習慣をたずねて No. と返答があったときに、なぜ No. なのかを聞きたい・聞く必要があるときに使います。

☐ 何かアレルギーはありますか。
　Do you have any allergies?

⇨ 日常の習慣をたずねるときには、現在形を用います。日本人として苦労するのが allergy の発音です。カタカナの「アレルギー」とは発音が違うので注意が必要です。

・・・ 患者の日常の習慣を聞く表現

喫煙
タバコは吸いますか。 **Do you smoke?**
1日に何本［何パック］吸いますか。
How many cigarettes [packs] a day?
＊タバコは通常 cigarette を使います。

飲酒
飲酒はなさいますか。 **Do you drink?**
ビール、ワイン、あるいは蒸留酒ですか。
Do you drink beer, wine or spirits?
通常どのくらい飲まれますか。
How much do you usually drink?

運動
規則的に運動をなさっていますか。
Do you exercise regularly?
1日に何時間くらいですか。
How many hours a day?

食事
バランスのよい食事をしていますか。
Do you eat a balanced diet?
規則的に食事をしていますか。
Do you eat regular meals? / Do you eat regulary?

睡眠
よく眠れますか。 **Do you sleep well?**
眠れなくて困ることはありますか。
Do you have trouble falling asleep?

ストレス
よくストレスを感じますか。 **Do you often get stressed?**
日頃、ストレスのある仕事をしていますか。
Do you usually work under stress?

その他
便通は規則正しいですか。
Do you have regular bowel movements?
生理は規則正しいですか。
Do you have regular menstrual periods?
他にあなたの体で気になっていることはありますか。
Do you have any other concerns about your body?
他に何か言っておきたいことはありますか。
Is there anything else you'd like to add?

● 会話例 1

Dr. Are you taking any medication?
何か薬を服用なさっていますか。

Pt. I've been taking cold medicine since the fever started.
熱が出てから、風邪薬を服用しています。

Dr. Are you taking any other drugs that we need to know about?
その他に何か私たちに話しておく必要のある薬を服用なさっていますか。

Pt. I can't think of anything in particular.
特にありません。

Dr. Do you have any allergies?
何かアレルギーはありますか。

Pt. No, I don't. I can eat anything.
いいえ、ありません。何でも食べられます。

● 会話例 2

Dr. Do you get a flu shot regularly?
規則的にインフルエンザの予防注射は受けていますか。

Pt. No, I don't.
いいえ、受けていません。

Dr. Is there any particular reason why not?
予防注射を受けないのには何か特別な理由がありますか。

Pt. Yeah, I have allergies, so my home doctor decided I shouldn't have one.
はい、私はアレルギーがあるので、かかりつけの先生が受けるべきではないと判断なさいました。

Dr. I see.
わかりました。

▶ flu shot：インフルエンザの予防注射

● 会話例 3

Dr. Do you smoke?
タバコはお吸いになりますか。

Pt. Yes.
はい。

Dr. How many cigarettes a day?
1日何本くらい吸いますか。

Pt. Well, I smoke at least one pack a day. I know it's not good for my health, though.
そうですねえ、1日に最低1箱は吸います。体によくないとはわかっているのですが。

Dr. Do you drink?
飲酒はなさいますか。

Pt. I'm a social drinker. I'm careful not to drink too much.
付き合い程度に飲みます。飲み過ぎないように心がけています。

＊ I'm a social drinker. は「私はパーティーなどの外出時のみ飲酒します」という意味です。

● 会話例 4

Dr. May I ask what your occupation is?
職業をお聞きしてもよろしいですか。

Pt. Yes, I'm an engineer.
はい、エンジニアです。

Dr. Has anything in your environment changed recently?
最近環境の変化がありましたか。

Pt. Yes, I was moved to another section in a personnel reshuffle.
はい、人事異動で別の部署へ移動になりました。

Dr. Would you say your work is pretty stressful?
仕事のストレスは多いですか。

Pt. I think so.
多いと思います。

Chapter 2 - 問診

4 既往歴・家族歴をたずねる

ここでは、患者の病気に関するバックグラウンドをたずねます。本人の病歴や家族の病歴となると、話しづらい患者もいる可能性があります。患者の不安を軽減するためにも、言葉を選んで丁寧にたずねていきます。

既往症をたずねる

- 病歴について少しお伺いできますか。
  Could you tell me a little bit about your medical history?

⇨ Could you tell me ～? という丁寧な言い方に、a little bit about ～を重ねます。

- 今まで何か大きな病気にかかったことがありますか。
  Have you ever had any serious illness?
- 薬に何かアレルギーがありますか。
  Have you ever had an allergic reaction to any medication?

⇨ 過去の病歴（経験）を聞くときは、現在完了形を使います。
Have you ever had any ～?（今までに何か～の経験がありますか）と聞かれた患者は、時期をはっきりさせる場合、When I was ... や 5 years ago などと過去形を使って答えます。

- 過去の病歴について教えてください。
  Tell me about any past illnesses.

⇨ このように、簡潔に聞くこともできます。

家族歴をたずねる

- ご家族でがんを患った方はいらっしゃいますか。
  ・Is there a history of cancer in your family?
  ・Does your family have a history of cancer?

⇨ 家族は、親、兄弟姉妹、叔父、叔母、祖父母を指し、患者本人の病歴情報にならない配偶者や子供は含まれません。

● 病名リスト

主な病名のリストです。五十音順にしてあります。
なお、それぞれの病名については、PART 2 で詳しく取り上げます。

悪性貧血	Pernicious Anemia
アルツハイマー病	Alzheimer's Disease
胃潰瘍	Ulcers; Peptic Ulcers; Gastic Ulcers
潰瘍性大腸炎	Ulcerative Colitis (UC)
インフルエンザ	Flu; Influenza
うつ病	Depression
関節リウマチ	Rheumatoid Arthritis (RA)
顔面神経痛	Facial Paralysis; Bell's Palsy
傷	Wounds
虚血性心疾患	Ischemic Heart Disease
高血圧症	High Blood Pressure; Hypertension
骨折	Fractures
痔核	Hemorrhoids; Piles
子宮筋腫	Fibroids; Myoma Uteri
歯根管	Root Canals
手根管症候群	Carpal Tunnel Syndrome
静脈瘤	Varicose Veins
神経痛	Nerve Pain
心臓疾患	Heart Disease
腎臓病	Kidney Disease; Kidney Failure
じんましん	Rashes
頭痛	Headache
摂食障害	Eating Disorders
ぜんそく	Asthma
前立腺肥大	Enlarged Prostate; Prostatic Hyperplasia
双極性障害	Bipolar Disorder
胆石	Gallstones; Cholelithiasis
虫垂炎	Appendicitis
できもの	Skin Tumors
てんかん	Epilepsy
糖尿病	Diabetes (Mellitus)
動脈硬化	Hardening of the Arteries; Arteriosclerosis
ドライアイ	Dry Eye Syndrome

乳腺腫瘍	Breast Growths
抜け毛	Hair Loss
ねんざ	Sprains
脳卒中	Stroke
白内障	Cataracts
鼻炎・副鼻腔炎	Sinus Infections; Rhinitis
皮下腫瘍	Subcutaneous Tumors
皮膚アレルギー	Skin Allergies
分娩	Childbirth
閉塞性睡眠時無呼吸	Obstructive Sleep Apnea (OSA)
ヘルニア	Hernia
弁膜症	Valvular Disease
膀胱炎	Cystitis
慢性閉塞性肺疾患	Chronic Obstructive Pulmonary Disease (COPD)
耳感染症	Ear Infections
メニエール病	Meniere's Disease
めまい・耳鳴り	Dizziness
腰痛	Backache
リンパ腫	Lymphoma

● 会話例 1

Dr. Could you tell me a little bit about your medical history?
病歴について少しお伺いできますか。

Pt. Yes, I was diagnosed with breast cancer 5 years ago. I was successfully treated at the time.
はい、私は5年前に乳がんと診断されました。その時、治療に成功しました。

Dr. Is there a history of cancer in your family?
ご家族でがんを患った方はいらっしゃいますか。

Pt. Yes, my father died of stomach cancer.
はい、父は胃がんで亡くなりました。

▶ be successfully treated：治療に成功する

会話例2

Dr. Have you ever had an allergic reaction to any food or medication?
食べ物や薬にアレルギーがありますか。

Pt. I'm allergic to dairy products.
乳製品にアレルギーがあります。

Dr. Has anyone in your family had the same issue?
ご家族で同じ問題を持っている方はいらっしゃいますか。

Pt. Yes, my younger sister has it, too.
はい、妹も同じアレルギーです。

雑学
Lay terms(一般用語)とProfessional terms(専門用語)

病気の症状や処置などを説明する言葉には2通りがあります。

professional termsは医師や科学者たちがお互いに用いる言葉ですが、専門的で一般の患者さんにはわかりにくいものです。そのため、医師がわかりやすく患者さんに説明に使うのがlay termsです。

日本語でも、「仰臥位」(professional terms)はわかりやすく言えば「仰向け」ですが、医師が学会でパワーポイントを示しながら説明すると、

「これは仰臥位(ぎょうがい)での患者の手術法です」

This is a surgical technique with the patient in the supine position.
となります。医師が患者に話す場合は、

「仰向けになってください」

"Please lie on your back." となります。

	Professional term(s)		Lay term(s)
1.	tumor; polyp	腫瘍、ポリープ	growth
2.	pulmonary issue	肺疾患	lung problem
3.	prophylaxis [prophylactic]	予防薬	(type of) drug that prevents disease or infection
4.	anemia [anemic]	貧血	iron deficiency (have) decreased red blood cells
5.	hematoma; contusion	血腫	bruise
6.	edema [edematous]	浮腫	swelling [be swollen]
7.	myocardial infarction	心臓発作	heart attack
8.	tibia	脛骨	shin
9.	respiration	呼吸	breathing

Chapter 3 - 身体診察

1 　視診・聴診・触診を行う ●●●

Chapter 2で取り上げた問診(Medical Interview)とともに、身体診察(Physical Examination)は患者の症状を的確に把握するうえで重要な情報源です。ここでは視診、聴診、触診に関わる会話を紹介します。

診察を始める

- ☐ 診察を始めましょう。
  - Let's take a look. / Let me take a look.
  - Let's have a look. / Let me have a look.

⇨ 「診察します」と言うときは、Let's ～「～しましょう」やLet me ～「～させてください」を使うと、一緒に診察を行うという気持ちが伝わり、患者の気持ちを和らげる助けになります。

服の着脱を指示する

- ☐ 上半身を脱いでください。
  Take off your clothes from the waist up.

- ☐ では、服を着ていただいていいですよ。
  You can get dressed now.

- ☐ 服を脱いでこのガウンを着てください。
  Take off your clothes and put this gown on.

- ☐ シャツを上に上げてください。
  Lift up your shirt.

⇨ 身体診察の指示は簡潔にするために、逐一pleaseをつけなくても構いません。ただし威圧的にならないように、言い方に気をつける必要があります。

体の向きを指示する

- ☐ 仰向け [うつ伏せ] になってください。
  Lie down on your back [stomach].

- ☐ 横向きになってください。
  Lie down on your side.

- ☐ 横向きでこちら［壁の方］を向いてください。
  Lie down on your side, facing me [the wall].

視診をする

- ☐ 両目だけで私の指を追ってください。
  Follow my finger just with your eyes.

⇨ 脳神経機能を見るための指示です。目だけで指の動きを追うように just with your eyes を使います。

- ☐ 左目［右目］を覆って。
  Cover your left [right] eye.
- ☐ まばたきをしないように。
  Try not to blink.
- ☐ 舌［目］を見せて。
  Let me see your tongue [eyes].
- ☐ 大きく口を開けて。
  Open your mouth wide.
- ☐ 口を開けて「アー」と言って。
  Open your mouth and say, "Ahhhhh."
- ☐ 舌を出して。
  Stick out your tongue.

聴診をする

- ☐ 呼吸の音を聞かせてください。
  Let me check your breathing.

⇨ 「心音を聞かせて」というときは Listen to your chest. と言います。

- ☐ 深呼吸をしてください。
  Take some deep breaths.

- ☐ 息を吸って[吐いて]。
  Breathe in [out].

⇨ レントゲンの撮影など、深呼吸が1回の場合はTake a deep breath. ですが、聴診では何度も深呼吸してもらう必要があるので、Take some deep breaths. と複数形にします。名詞はbreath、動詞はbreatheと発音の違いも要注意です。

触診をする

- ☐ 腕[肩／腹]の力を抜いてください。
  Relax your arms [shoulders / stomach].

⇨ 力を抜いて楽にしてもらいたいときはrelaxを使いますが、患者の力が抜けるよう、柔らかい口調で言う必要があります。両腕の力を抜いてほしいときは、Relax your arms. と複数形になります。

- ☐ ここを押すと[触ると／たたくと]痛みますか。
  Does it hurt when I press [touch / tap] here?

⇨ 触診の際に痛みを感じる部位を教えてもらうときの表現です。

- ☐ ここが痛かったら言ってください。
  Tell me if this hurts.

- ☐ ここは痛くないでしょう。
  This won't hurt.

- ☐ ここは少し痛いかもしれません。
  This may hurt a bit.

- ☐ ここはどうですか。
  How about here?

会話例 1　視診

Dr. Please look straight at the spot on the wall.
あの壁のあの点をまっすぐ見てください。

Pt. Like this?
これでよろしいですか。

Dr. Good. I'm going to shine a light in your eyes. Try not to blink.
はい。これから目に光を当てます。まばたきをしないようにしてください。

Dr. OK.
結構です。

会話例 2　聴診

Dr. Let me check your breathing. Please take off your shirt and sit up on the examining table.
呼吸を調べましょう。シャツを脱いで、診察台にお座りください。

Pt. OK.
わかりました。

Dr. Good. Now, I'm going to press the stethoscope against your back and listen.
結構ですよ。これから背中に聴診器を当てて呼吸音を聞きます。

会話例 3　触診

Dr. I'd like to take a look at your stomach. Please lie down on your back on the exam table.
お腹を診せてください。診察台の上で仰向けになってください。

Pt. Is this all right?
これでいいですか。

Dr. Yes, you're fine. Just relax. Does it hurt when I press here?
はい、結構です。力を抜いてください。ここを押すと痛みますか。

Pt. ... aah!
あいたたた。

Chapter 3 身体診察

2 バイタルサインの評価を行う

身体診察では、視診、触診、聴診などによる全身状態の把握のほか、バイタルサイン（脈拍、呼吸、体温、血圧等）の評価を行います。ここでは、脈拍、体温、血圧などを測る際の表現を紹介します。

脈拍・血圧を測る

- ☐ 脈拍［血圧］を測りましょう。
  Let's take your pulse [blood pressure].

- ☐ 脈拍を測らせてください。
  Let me feel your pulse.

- ☐ 血圧を測らせてください。
  Let me measure your blood pressure.

⇨ 「脈」は pulse または pulse rate です。「脈を測る」は take だけでなく、feel someone's pulse と feel も使えます。

- ☐ 脈拍は80です。
  Your pulse is 80 beats per minute.

- ☐ 血圧は上が150で下が110です。
  Your blood pressure is 150 over 110.

⇨ 血圧の値は、収縮期血圧（高い方）と拡張期血圧（低い方）の間に over を入れて表現します。脈拍や血圧はその数値が、患者の緊張の度合いによって左右される場合があります。できるだけリラックスした状態で測定するため、Just relax.（リラックスしてください）、Take it easy.（心配ありません）、You're doing fine.（いいですよ）といった声かけをしていくのもよい方法です。

体温を測る

- ☐ 熱を測りましょう。
  Let's take your temperature.

- ☐ 熱があるかどうか見てみましょう。
  Let's see if you have a temperature.

⇨ 摂氏36度5分 (thirty-six point five degrees Centigrade) は、華氏だと97.7度 (ninety-seven point seven degrees Fahrenheit) です。米国は華氏表記です。

体温の測り方

測定する部位ごとに検温に必要な時間や方法が異なり、測定値も異なります。また、日本ではわきの下での検温が主流ですが、検温方法は国によっても異なります。

鼓膜電子体温計（Tympanic Electronic）

…… 耳に入れて体温を測ります。痛くありませんし、数秒で終わります。

We'll use this electronic thermometer, which is inserted in your ear. It doesn't hurt and will take only a few seconds.

口腔内電子体温計（Oral Electronic）

…… 舌の裏側に入れて測ります。音が鳴るまで待ってください。

Hold this electronic thermometer under your tongue. Wait until the thermometer beeps.

腋窩で測音（Axillary）

…… わきの下で体温を測ります。（次頁の「会話例３ 体温」参照）

肛門で測温（Rectal）

…… 一番正確に体温を測るためにお尻の穴から体温を測ります。診察台の上に脇腹を下にするようにして横に寝てください。服を下げてください。少し気持ちが悪いかもしれません。体温を測るまでに数分かかります。

In order to get the most accurate reading, we need to check your temperature rectally. Lie down here on the examining table on your side and lower your clothes. This may be a little uncomfortable. It will take a few minutes to register.

● 会話例１　脈拍　

N I'd like to take your pulse. Let me have your wrist.
脈拍を測らせてください。手首を診ましょう。

Pt. Do you need me to do something?
私が何かする必要はありますか。

N No … just breathe normally and relax … Your pulse is normal … It's 80 beats per minute.
いいえ、ただ普通にリラックスして呼吸をしてください。脈拍は正常です。１分間に80です。

● 会話例 2　血圧

N Let's check your blood pressure. Hold out your arm and make a fist. The cuff might pinch a little but try to hold still.
血圧を測りましょう。腕を出して、手を握ってください。少しきつくて痛いかもしれませんが動かないでください。

N Your blood pressure is 150 over 110. Do you usually have hypertension?
血圧は上が150で下が110です。普段から血圧は高い方ですか。

Pt. No, it's usually normal. I think I'm a little nervous today.
いいえ、普段は普通です。今日は少し緊張しているのかもしれません。

● 会話例 3　体温

N Have you taken your temperature this morning?
今朝、熱を測りましたか。

Pt. No, I haven't.
いいえ。

N Let's take your temperature. Please put this thermometer under your arm.
熱を測りましょう。体温計をわきの下にはさんでください。

N Your temperature is 38 degrees Centigrade. That's 100.4 degrees Fahrenheit.
摂氏38度。華氏にすると100.4度です。

● 会話例 4　体重

N Has your weight changed recently?
最近、体重に変化はありますか。

Pt. I've actually lost 10 pounds in the past two weeks.
実は2週間で10ポンド減りました。

N Hmm, so you've lost about 5 kilos. Let's weigh you now. Take off your shoes and stand on the scale over there.
なるほど、約5キロ減ったのですね。では体重を測りましょう。靴を脱いで、あそこの体重計にのってください。

Measurements
単位換算

Height …… 身長

インチとセンチメートル …… 1 inch → 2.54 cm

フィートとメートル …… 1 foot → 0.3 m (30cm)

Weight …… 体重

ポンドとキログラム …… 1 pound → 0.45 kg

　　　　　　　　　　　　1 kg → 2.2 pounds

例) 160 cm　56 kg → 5 feet 3 inches 123.4 pounds

　　175 cm　78 kg → 5 feet 9 inches 172.0 pounds

Body Temperature …… 体温

摂氏　Centigrade / Celsius

華氏　Fahrenheit

　　　　　華氏の換算値

0℃　→　32.0°F
35℃　→　95.0°F
36℃　→　96.8°F
37℃　→　98.6°F
39℃　→　102.2°F
40℃　→　104.0°F

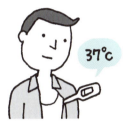
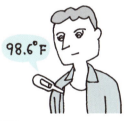

Pulse …… 脈拍

例) 脈拍68/秒 → sixty-eight beats per minute

Blood Pressure …… 血圧

高血圧　hypertension

低血圧　hypotension

例) 上が170で下が80 → 170 over 80

Chapter 4 - 検査

1 検査を指示する

採血や尿検査といった一般的な検査から精密検査に至るまで、病院ではさまざまな検査が行われますが、ここでは医師が患者に検査を指示する表現を紹介します。

検査を促す

☐ 検査室に行って血液検査をしていただきます。
I'm going to send you over to the lab for some blood tests.

⇨ send ~ over to ... は「~を…に送る[行かせる(行ってもらう)]」という意味で、医師が「検査を指示する」ときによく用いられます。

☐ いくつか検査をします。
I'm going to order some tests.

☐ いくつか検査をする必要があります。
We need to run some tests.

☐ あなたはいくつかの検査を受ける必要があります。
You need to have some tests.

⇨ 医師が「検査を行う」というときには order、run が用いられます。

☐ いくつか簡単な血液検査から始めたいと思います。
I'd like to start with some simple bloodwork.

☐ 念のため MRI 検査をします。
I'm going to order an MRI to find out for sure.

⇨ for sure は「確実に」という意味で、「確実に見つけるために」という意味です。

▶ bloodwork:「血液検査」(= blood test)

検査を行う理由を説明する

☐ 可能性のある問題点を取り除いていきたいので、いくつかの検査をしていきましょう。
I'd like to rule out some possible problems, so I'm going to order some tests.

- ☐ 感染症を頻繁に起こしているので、異常があるかどうかチェックしたいと思います。

  Because of the frequent infections, I'd like to check for a possible abnormality.

⇨ 「なぜ検査を受けなければならないのか」。これは患者さんにとって大いに気になることです。患者の不安を払拭するためにも、丁寧にわかりやすい説明を心がける必要があります。理由を述べるには so、because、because of などを用います。

- ☐ 狭心症の可能性があるので、胸のＸ線と心電図の手配から始めたいと思います。

  This could be angina. So I'd like to start by ordering a chest X-ray and an EKG.

⇨ could は「〜もありうる」と婉曲に可能性を述べます。
  - ▶ angina：狭心症

患者を落ち着かせる

- ☐ （検査結果を見て）そこから治療方針を考えましょう。

  We'll see where to go from there.

⇨ 症状に不安を感じる患者は少しでも早く結論を求めがちです。落ち着いてもらえるよう誠実に声をかけることが重要です。
  where to go は「どこへ進めばいいのか、どうすればいいのか」という意味ですから、医師と患者がどうすればいいのか（＝治療方針をどうすればいいのか）ということになります。

- ☐ 結論を急がないようにしましょう。

  Let's not jump to conclusions.

- ☐ いくつか検査を行うまでは、私たちがこれから何に取り組んでいくべきか具体的にはわかりません。

  Until we do some tests, we won't know exactly what we're dealing with.

検査手順・必要書類を指示する

☐ 検査前日の午後8時以降は一切飲食をしないでください。
Do not eat or drink anything after 8 pm the night before the test.

☐ 検査日の朝は何も食べないでください。
Nothing can be consumed on the morning of the test.

⇨ 検査手順は簡潔にわかりやすく説明します。

☐ この同意書に署名して、検査の当日にお持ちください。
Please sign this consent form and bring it with you on the day of the test.

☐ 受付で渡される検査書類を検査室へ持って行ってください。
Just take the paperwork that they'll give you at the desk to the laboratory.

▶ consent form：同意書

● 会話例 1

Dr. I'm going to send you over to the lab for some blood tests. Let's get a urine sample, as well.
これから検査室に行って血液検査をしていただきます。尿検査も行いましょう。

Pt. OK.
わかりました。

Dr. I'm going to put a rush on the labs and we'll see where to go from there.
検査を急がせますので、そこから治療方針を検討しましょう。

● 会話例 2

Dr. I'd like to rule out some possible problems, so I'm going to order some tests.
可能性のある問題点を取り除いていきたいので、検査をしていきましょう。

Pt. Could you explain what that involves?
どんな検査を行うのかを、説明していただけますか。

Dr. Sure. The stool sample will let us rule out bacteria, parasites or viruses. The blood tests will give us even more information.
もちろんです。便のサンプルを検査することで、細菌や寄生虫やウイルスがあなたの症状に関わりがないかどうかを判別できます。血液検査をすればもっと情報が得られるでしょう。

Pt. I see.
なるほど。

● 会話例 3

Pt. How much will this test cost?
この検査はいくらくらいかかりますか。

Dr. I think that part of the cost will be covered by your health insurance, so it should be around 5,000 yen.
あなたの加入している健康保険で一部カバーされると思いますので、5千円くらいでしょう。

● 会話例 4

Pt. I know this is a serious symptom that may indicate renal failure.
私にはこれが、腎不全を意味する深刻な症状だとわかっています。

Dr. Let's not jump to conclusions. I'd like to do some blood and urine tests and determine what's going on first.
結論を急がないようにしましょう。まず血液検査と尿検査を行って、あなたの症状を判断したいと思います。

● 会話例 5

N Please sign this consent form and bring it with you on the day of the test.
この同意書に署名して、検査の当日にお持ちください。

Pt. OK, sure.
わかりました、持参します。

N Is it possible to have someone accompany you?
どなたか付き添いの方に来てもらうことはできますか。

Pt. I'll try to ask a friend.
友人に頼もうと思います。

Chapter 4 — 検査

2　採血・尿検査をする

自国とは勝手も違い、外国人患者は日本の病院で行う検査に不安を感じるはずです。安心して検査が受けられるように、それぞれの手順において、事前の一言が必要です。ここでは基本的な検査である採血と尿検査に関わる表現を紹介します。

採血を指示する

- 採血をしましょう。
  Let's take a blood sample.

- 血液検査を行います。
  We'll do a blood test.

- 検査室で検査をしてもらうために採血を行う必要があります。
  I need to take a blood sample to send to the lab for some tests.

⇨ 「採血する」という表現にはtake blood、take a blood sampleなどがあります。ただしtake bloodは文字通り「血を取る」という意味で直接的過ぎるので、take a blood sampleを使った方がやわらかい表現になります。

患者の名前を確認する

- お名前を再確認させてください。
  We need to double-check your name.

⇨ 外国人患者の名前のスペリングの確認は難しいものです。患者本人に確認してもらうのが一番正確です。採血管に貼ってあるラベルを指し示し、Is your name correct?（あなたの名前で間違いありませんか）とたずねれば確実です。

採血前の指示

- ここに腕を置いていただけますか。
  Would you rest your arm here?

- 左[右]の腕を伸ばしてください。
  Hold out your left [right] arm.

- 袖をまくってください。
  Roll up your sleeve.

2 採血・尿検査をする

- ☐ 親指を中にして手を握ってください。
  Make a fist with your thumb inside.
- ☐ 手を2、3回強く握ってください。
  Squeeze your hand a few times.

⇨ make a fist は「こぶしをつくる」という意味。「固く握る」という場合は make a tight fist、「軽く握る」という場合は make a fist not so tight と言います。

- ☐ 少しチクッとするかもしれません。
  You might feel a little prick.
- ☐ 少し痛むかもしれません。
  You'll feel just a little pinch.

⇨ このように断っておくと、患者は心の準備ができるものです。little prick（チクチク痛む）や pinch（つねる）は hurt や pain ほどの大きな痛みを連想させません。

採血中に

- ☐ すぐに終わります。
  ・It will be finished in no time.
  ・We're almost done.
- ☐ 手を開き、楽にしてください。
  Open your hand up and relax.

⇨ 採血中、リラックスさせるためにこのように声をかけます。

- ☐ 血が止まるまで、これ（カット綿）で押さえてください。
  Press down on this until the bleeding stops.
- ☐ ここを数分間押さえていてください。
  ・Please apply pressure here for a few minutes.
  ・Please put some pressure on this for a few minutes.

⇨ 採血の後の処置を指示する表現です。

尿検査を指示する

- [ ] コップのこの線まで入れてください。
  Please fill the cup to this line.

- [ ] この線のところまでコップに尿を取ってきてください。
  Please fill this cup to the line with urine.

- [ ] 途中の尿を取ってきてください。
  Please collect the urine in mid-stream.

⇨ in mid-stream は中間尿の採取を指示する場合の言い方です。

● 会話例 1

N I need to get a blood sample. First, we need to double-check your name. Is this correct?
採血をいたします。まず、お名前を再確認させてください。これで間違いないですね。

Pt. Yes.
はい。

N Have you ever felt ill during a blood test? Have you ever developed a rash from rubbing alcohol?
採血中に気分が悪くなったことはありますか。消毒用のアルコールでかぶれたことはありますか。

Pt. No, I haven't had either issue.
いいえ、どちらもありませんでした。

N Okay. Would you rest your arm here? You might feel a little prick.
結構です。ここに腕を置いていただけますか。少しチクっとするかもしれません。

Pt. Uhm... all right.
え、はい。

N Let me know if there's any tingling or numbness.
何かうずくような痛みやしびれがあったら教えてください。

▶ develop a rash：かぶれる

2 採血・尿検査をする

● 会話例2

N We're almost done. Open your hand and relax.
もうすぐ終わります。手を開いて楽にしてください。

Pt Sure.
わかりました。

N All done. Please put some pressure on this for the next five minutes.
これで終わりです。ここを5分間押さえていてください。

● 会話例3

N Now we'd like to get a urine sample. There's a men's room around the corner to the left.
では、尿検査をします。男子トイレはその角を曲がった左手にあります。

―検尿用の紙コップを渡しながら―

N Please fill the cup to this line. Go ahead and leave the cup on the shelf inside and wash your hands.
（尿を）コップのこの線まで入れてください。コップはトイレの中の棚に置き、手を洗ってください。

Pt Okay. Thank you.
わかりました。ありがとう。

N When you get back, please have a seat here until you're called.
戻られたら、呼ばれるまでここにおかけになっていてください。

表現のポイント

トイレの英語表現

女性用トイレは ladies' room、男性用トイレは men's room が、丁寧かつ一般的で、どこの国でも用いられている表現です。共用トイレであっても使うことができます。

lavatory や bathroom も丁寧でよく使われる表現ですが、女性用か男性用かどちらを指すのかわからないのが難点です。また bathroom はもともと浴室を意味する語なので、米国人以外はこの表現を使用するのに違和感を持つことがあります。

Chapter 4 - 検査

3 さまざまな検査をする ●●●

ここでは、画像検査などのさまざまな機器を使った検査の言い方と、検査を受けてもらうときに必要な表現を見ていきましょう。

検査をする

☐ 胸のレントゲンを撮ります。
　We need to do a chest X-ray.
　I'd like to do a chest X-ray.

⇨ do a/an ～ (test) を使って、いろいろな検査の実行を患者に伝えることができます。
「検査をする」は、do 以外に take や have を使うことができます。
　We'll **take** an X-ray (of your arm).
　We'll **have** an X-ray (of your chest).

---

do a/an ～（test）
検査を表す言い方

聴力検査をする	do a hearing test
心電図をとる	do an EKG [ECG]
骨密度検査をする	do a bone density test
肺機能検査をする	do a lung function test
レントゲン検査をする	do an X-ray
超音波検査をする	do an ultrasound
MRI 検査をする	do an MRI
内視鏡検査をする	do an endoscopic exam [test]
CT スキャンをする	do a CT (scan)

＊ X-ray, ultrasound, MRI (magnetic resonance imaging), endoscopic はいずれも最初が母音なので冠詞は an になります。EKG, MRI, CT はいずれも略語で言った方がわかりやすいでしょう。また、心電図はドイツ語の Elektrokardiogramm が語源で、ほとんどの場合、略語の EKG が用いられます。（ECG は electrocardiogram の略）

3 さまざまな検査をする

> □ 息を深く吸って、そのまま止めてください。
> Take a deep breath in and hold it.

⇨ 「息を吸う・吐く」の表現は、take a breath in [out] のほかにも、breathe in [out] や inhale [exhale] があります。breath [bréθ] と breathe [bríːð] の発音の違いは要注意です。

● 会話例 1　レントゲン　　　　　　　　　　

T We need to do a chest X-ray. Is there any chance you might be pregnant?
胸のレントゲンを撮ります。妊娠している可能性はありますか。

Pt. No.
いいえ。

T OK. Please wait here.
了解です。ここでお待ちください。

Pt. Sure.
はい。

T (Technician): Please come in, take off your shirt and put on this gown. Please remove any metallic accessories. If your bra has metal hooks, please take that off, too.
中に入って、まずシャツを脱ぎ、このガウンに着替えてください。金属類は取ってください。ブラジャーに金属のフックが付いていれば、それも外してください。

Pt. OK.
はい。

T Now stand here and turn this way.
ではここに立って、こちらを向いてください。

T Next, I'd like you to breathe in deeply and hold your breath.
次に息を深く吸って、そのまま息を止めてください。

T Very good.
大変結構です。

● **会話例2　バリウム検査**

T We want to do a GI series which is a type of X-ray that'll show your stomach and upper intestine. After you get undressed, you'll be escorted to the fluoroscopy room.
これから胃と小腸のレントゲン検査を行います。支度を終えられたら透視検査室にご案内します。

Pt. I'm ready.
用意ができました。

T Now, I need you to drink this barium.
では、このバリウムをお飲みください。

Pt. OK.
はい。

T I'll use the fluoroscope to watch how the barium goes down after you swallow it. I'll also take some X-rays from time to time.
バリウムを飲んだあと、それが体の中を通る様子を透視して確認します。その途中で何枚かレントゲン写真も撮ります。

T I'll be asking you to move into various positions on the X-ray table. The whole procedure takes about 15 minutes.
レントゲン台の上で、いろいろな姿勢をとっていただきます。検査は15分ほどかかります。

▶ fluoroscopy room：透視検査室

● **会話例3　エコー（超音波検査）**

T We need to do an ultrasound. Please lie down here.
超音波検査をします。ここに横になってください。

Pt. Okay.
はい。

T Could you please bend your knees?
膝を曲げていただけますか。

Pt. Like this?
このようにですか。

T Good. Now, I'm going to apply a gel to your stomach. It's going to feel a little cool.
結構です。では、このジェルをお腹に塗ります。少し冷たく感じます。

T Take a deep breath in and expand your stomach. Hold it.
大きく息を吸ってお腹を膨らませてください。息を止めてください。

T You can relax now. ... Okay, would you turn onto your left side?
では、楽にしてください。結構です。左向きに横になっていただけますか。

T Good. Now, turn on your back.
結構です。では、仰向けに戻ってください。

T We're almost done. I'm just going to clean up your abdomen with a warm towel.
あともう少しです。ちょっと温かいタオルでお腹を拭きますね。

＊最後に看護師が温かいタオルで患者のお腹を拭いていますが、これは外国ではあまり行われないサービスなので、事前に「温かいタオルでお腹を拭きます」と断りを入れてから行っています。

● 会話例4　心電図　

T We need to do an EKG. I'd like you to lie down here.
心電図をとります。ここに横になってください。

Pt. Okay.
はい。

T Would you take off your socks and pull up your shirt?
靴下を脱いで、シャツを上に上げてくださいますか。

T I need you to keep still while the EKG is being taken.
心電図をとっている間は、動かないようにしてください。

T It takes about 10 minutes to complete this test.
検査はだいたい10分くらいで終わります。

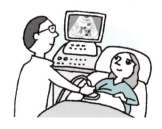

● 会話例 5　乳房 X 線撮影　

T We need to get a mammogram. This machine will press on your breast. It might be little uncomfortable.
マンモグラフィー検査を行います。この機械で胸を挟みます。少し痛いかもしれません。

Pt. OK.
わかりました。

T If you can't stand the discomfort, please let me know.
我慢できなかったら教えてください。

T We'll start with your left breast. Please put your feet on this line, and place your breast here.
では、左から撮ります。この線のところに立って、胸をここにのせてください。

T Hold still.
このまま動かないでください。

T Now I need you to breathe in and then hold your breath.
では、息を吸ったまま止めてください。

Pt. Ouch!
痛い！

T Are you all right?
大丈夫ですか。

Pt. Yeah ...
ええ…

T We're done with the tests for today. We'll let you know the test results in about two weeks. Thank you for your patience.
これで今日の検査はすべて終了です。検査結果は約 2 週間後にお伝えします。お疲れさまでした。

Pt. Thank you.
ありがとうございました。

▶ **uncomfortable**：不快な ＊患者の不安感を取り除くには、painful や hurt といった「痛み」を連想する語はできるだけ使わないほうがよいでしょう。そういった場合に uncomfortable や discomfort を使います。

discomfort：不快感

Thank you for your patience.：お疲れ様でした。＊相手を待たせたり、痛みを伴う検査を終えたときなどに使うと有効です。

● 検査名リスト

一般的な検査	Common Tests
喀痰検査	sputum test
血液検査	blood test
検便	stool test
心電図	EKG (Elektrokardiogramm)
超音波検査	ultrasound
聴力検査	hearing test
尿検査	urinalysis
脳波検査	EEG (Electroencephalogram)
肺機能検査	lung function test
胸部レントゲン	chest X-ray
眼の検査	eye test

精密検査		Detailed Tests	
胃内視鏡検査		gastroscopy	
気管支鏡検査		bronchoscopy	
骨塩定量測定検査		BMD (Bone Mineral Density)	
骨密度検査		bone density test	
CTスキャン	コンピュータ断層撮影	CT Scan	Computerized Tomography
サーモグラフィー		thermography	
磁気共鳴映像法		MRI (Magnetic Resonance Imaging)	
大腸内視鏡検査		colonoscopy	
内視鏡検査		endoscopy	
パップ試験	子宮がん検査法	pap test	uterine cancer screening
バリウム注腸	下部消化器造影	barium enema	lower GI series
バリウム粥	上部消化器造影	barium meal	upper GI series
腹腔鏡検査		laparoscopy	
膀胱鏡検査		cystoscopy	
乳房X線撮影		mammogram [mammography]	
腰椎穿刺		spinal tap	

Chapter 5 — 診断・処置・処方

1　検査結果を伝える

検査結果の報告を受け、患者に結果を伝えます。結果が芳しくない場合でも、患者がうろたえたり、落ち込んだりしないようにしながら、結果を正確に伝える必要があります。

検査結果を伝える — 最初のフレーズ

- ☐ こちらが検査結果です。
  - ・Here's what we found out.
  - ・Here are your test results.

⇨ 検査結果を患者に伝えるときには、検査画像が映し出されたり、検査結果の数値が記された書類を手元に置いての会話となります。そのため、Here's 〜、Here are 〜といった表現が使われます。なお、結果を意味する result は通常、複数形 results で使います。

- ☐ 検査結果をご説明しましょう。
  - ・Let me explain your test results.
  - ・I'd like to explain your test results.

検査結果を伝える — よい結果の場合

- ☐ 検査の結果は正常です。
  - ・The test shows that everything is normal.
  - ・According to the tests, everything looks normal.

⇨ ここでも検査結果を見ながらの会話なので、show（〜を示す）や look（〜のように見える）が用いられます。

- ☐ 検査の結果によると、あなたは糖尿病ではないと思います。
  According to the results, I don't believe you have diabetes.

- ☐ 検査によると何も問題はありません。
  According to the test, you have no problem.

⇨ 検査の結果をもとに説明するときには according to 〜「〜によると」を使います。

□ 何も心配はないようです。
　It looks like you don't have anything to worry about.

□ 胃はきれいに見えます。
　・Your stomach looks healthy.
　・Your stomach looks very good.

⇨ look を使って表現をやわらかくすることができます。It looks like (that) ... は「…のように見える」という意味です。

検査結果を伝える—悪い結果の場合

□ 残念ながら、検査の結果はあなたが結腸のがんであることを示しています。
　I'm sorry to say that your test results indicate that you have a cancer in the colon.

⇨ I'm sorry to say that ... や I'm sorry to have to tell you that ... を使って「残念ですが…と言わなければなりません」と断って結果を伝えます。あるいは、We have a small problem.「少し問題があります」と最初に断ってから、検査結果を伝えることもできます。

□ 検査結果は、あなたの肝臓の左側に悪性腫瘍があることを示しています。
　The test results show that you have a malignant tumor in the left side of your liver.

□ 胸部のX線検査の結果によると、あなたは肺疾患の状態にあるようです。
　Based on your chest X-rays, it looks like you have a lung condition.

⇨ show は test results を主語とし「～を示唆する、意味する」という意味を表します。indicate、suggest や it を主語にして It looks like ...「…のようだ」を使うこともできます。

数値の問題を伝える

□ 血液検査の結果によると、白血球数が高くなっています。
　According to the blood test, your white blood cell count is high.

⇨ 検査結果の数値に問題がある場合、is high [low]「高い[低い]」、is a little high [low]「少し高い[低い]」、is rather high [low]「かなり高い[低い]」といった表現を使います。

以下の表現も使えます。
You have a high [low] white blood cell count.
Your white blood cell count has increased [decreased].

- ☐ 血液検査によると、白血球がかなり増えています。
  Your blood test indicates that your white blood cell count is rather high.

- ☐ 血液検査によると、血糖値が高めになっています。
  Your blood test shows that your blood sugar level has become higher.

- ☐ 検査結果はあなたの血糖値とコレステロール値が高いことを示しています。
  Your test results indicate that your blood sugar and cholesterol are high.

- ☐ 超音波検査でいくつか胆嚢に石が見つかりました。
  The ultrasound showed several stones in your gallbladder.

再検査を伝える

- ☐ 念のため、もう一度血液検査をしましょう。
  Let us do another blood test to be sure.

- ☐ 血液検査をもう一度行いたいと思います。
  I'd like to get another blood test.

- ☐ CTスキャンをもう一度撮りましょう。
  We'll need to get another CT scan.

⇨ 「もう一度」という場合、名詞を修飾する場合にはanotherを使って、do another test、get another testといった形にします。

- ☐ 念のため、生検をもう一度する必要があります。
  We'll need to repeat the biopsy to be sure.

⇨ 動詞repeatを使って言うこともできます。

1 検査結果を伝える

● 会話例 1

Dr. Here's what we found out. We have a small problem. Your test shows that your white blood cell count is rather high.
これが検査結果です。少々問題があります。血液検査によると、白血球がかなり増えています。

Pt. What does that mean?
それはどういう意味ですか。

Dr. It means that there's probably inflammation somewhere in your body.
あなたの身体の中のどこかで炎症が起こっている可能性があるということです。

● 会話例 2

Dr. I'm looking at the results of your hemoglobin A1C test and you're quite a bit higher than normal. I believe you have diabetes.
ヘモグロビンA1C検査の結果を拝見しているところですが、正常よりもかなり高いですね。あなたは糖尿病だと思います。

Pt. Does this mean I have to stop eating sweets?
私は甘いものを食べるのをやめなければならないということでしょうか。

Dr. Diabetes is a more complicated disease than you think. Let me explain a bit further.
糖尿病はあなたが考えておられるよりももっと複雑な症状です。もう少し詳しく説明しましょう。

● 会話例 3

Dr. Based on your biopsy, you have a cancer in the right lung.
生検の結果、右の肺にがんが見つかりました。

Pt. Oh, no.
ええっ、そんな。

Dr. If we find that the disease is limited to the one area where we took the biopsy, it will mean that this is still in Stage 1. We'd like to get another biopsy to be sure.
病状が生検で採取した1カ所に限られていれば、これはまだ第1ステージだということです。念のため、生検をもう一度行いましょう。

Chapter 5 - 診断・処置・処方
2　処方箋を出す

診察や検査結果にもとづいて処方箋を出します。ここでは、処方箋に関わる表現を紹介します。

処方箋を出す場合

☐ 抗生物質を処方します。
　I'm going to prescribe an antibiotic.

⇨ prescribe「処方する」と prescription「処方箋」と医師・薬剤師・患者の関係は次のようになります。
医師は患者のために薬を処方する。
A doctor **prescribes** medicine for the patient.
薬剤師は患者のために処方薬を調合する。
A pharmacist fills the **prescription** for the patient.
患者は処方された薬を服用する。
The patient takes the **prescribed** medicine.

処方箋を出さない場合

☐ 今日は薬は出ません。
　You don't need to get the medicine today.

⇨ you を主語にして don't need to get で言うことができます。

薬の説明

☐ これは高血圧を治療する薬です。ほとんど副作用を起こす人はいませんが、めまいを起こす人もいます。
　It is used to treat high blood pressure. Most people have no side effects but sometimes it can cause dizziness.

⇨ it is used to treat ～「～を治療するのに使われます」で薬の目的を説明しています。
　▶ side effect：副作用　　dizziness：めまい

☐ この処方箋を薬局に提出してください。病院内でも病院外でも結構です。
　You can submit this prescription either to the pharmacy inside the hospital or to one outside.

⇨ submit the prescription to ～で「処方箋を～に提出する」という意味になります。

- ☐ 1ヶ月分処方して様子を見たいと思います。
  I'd like to give it a month and see how you do.

- ☐ 1ヶ月分処方しますから、様子を見ましょう。
  Why don't we give it a month and see how you do?

⇨ 処方箋を出すと同時に、患者に日常生活で気を付けなければならないことを伝えます。

日常生活のアドバイスを行う

- ☐ 私が処方した薬に加えて、ふだんの食事に注意していただきたいと思います。
  In addition to the medication that I've prescribed, I'd like you to watch your diet.

- ☐ これをしばらく服用していただいて、経過観察をします。
  We're going to have you take them for a while and monitor your progress.

- ☐ この新しい薬がどう作用するか見たいので、2、3週間したらまた受診してください。
  I'd like to see you again in two to three weeks to see how you're doing on this new medication.

- ☐ 当分の間、アスピリンも止めることもお勧めします。
  I also suggest that you lay off the aspirin for the time being.

- ☐ 乳製品の摂取も制限するべきです。
  You should also limit your dairy intake.

- ☐ 副作用の可能性がありますので、何か問題があれば直ちに連絡してください。
  There can be side effects, so I want you to let me know immediately if you have any issues.

- ☐ この薬によって通常より尿の回数が増えるかもしれません。
  This medicine may cause you to urinate more frequently than usual.

- ☐ 5日分の胃薬も処方します。これは単に予防措置です。
  I'm also prescribing five days of stomach medicine. This is just a precaution.

会話例 1

Dr. I'm going to prescribe something a bit milder that should have a similar effect on the pain.
痛みに対して同様の効果を持つもう少し穏やかなものを処方しましょう。

Pt. What kind of medication is this?
それはどんな薬ですか。

Dr. It's a combination drug that includes two types of painkillers. I'd like to give it a month and see how you do.
これは2種類の鎮痛剤を含んだ配合剤です。1ヶ月分処方して、様子を見たいと思います。

Pt. All right. Thank you.
わかりました。ありがとうございます。

会話例 2

Dr. Why don't you start out by taking two of these lozenges per day and see if you begin to feel better?
このトローチ剤の1日2錠の服用を開始して、具合がよくなり始めるか様子を見ましょう。

Pt. It doesn't sound so serious if we're treating it with lozenges.
トローチで治るのなら、それほど深刻な症状ではないようですね。

Dr. True. I don't think you have to worry about this right now. However, I'd like to see you again in three to four weeks.
そうですね。現段階で症状のことを心配する必要はないと思います。でも3、4週間後にもう一度診察させてください。

▶ lozenge：トローチ剤

薬の服用法を説明する表現

種類 ………… 飲んでいただくのはカプセルと錠剤で数種類あります。
There are several kinds of capsules and tablets to take.

何日分 ……… 5日分の薬です。
This is enough medicine for five days.

薬を飲むとき … 〜を感じたときに、これらの錠剤を2錠服用してください。
If you feel 〜, take two of these tablets.

痛いとき ……………… If you feel pain,

かゆいとき ……………… If you feel itchy,

胸が苦しいとき ……… If you feel pressure in the chest,

眠れないとき……………… If it is hard to sleep,

熱が38.5度以上あるとき …… If your temperature is over 38.5℃,

保管 ……… 薬は冷蔵庫で保管してください。
Keep the medicine in the refrigerator.

飲み方 ……… 熱いお湯で溶かして飲んでください。
Dissolve it with hot water and drink.
これは原液ですので2倍に薄めて使ってください。
This is an undiluted solution so please mix one part medicine with two parts (water) before you take it.

服用する量 ……1回1目盛りずつ飲んでください。
Drink the marked portion of it at one time.
1日3回、食後［食前］に飲んでください。
Take it three times a day after meals [before meals].
朝食と夕食後に2錠ずつ飲んでください。
Take two tablets after breakfast and after dinner.
6時間おきに2錠ずつ飲んでください。
Take two tablets every six hours.

坐薬・軟膏 …… これは坐薬です。肛門から入れてください。
This is a suppository. Please insert it anally.
この軟膏を痛むところに塗ってください。
Apply this ointment where you feel pain.

注意事項 …… 使用方法を注意深く読んでください。
Read the directions carefully.
尿の色が変わるかもしれませんが心配ありません。
The color of your urine may change, but don't worry.
眠くなりますので、車の運転や危険な作業は避けてください。
Avoid driving and using heavy machinery because this medicine will make you sleepy.

Chapter 5 - 診断・処置・処方

3 次の予約を入れる

診察の最後に、再診が必要な患者に対して、次の診察日を調整して予約を入れます。ここでは、診察日と入院・手術など予約に関わる表現を見ていきます。

都合のよい日を伝える

- ☐ 1週間後に診察を受けに来ていただけますか。11月13日の月曜日です。
  Can you come back to see me a week from today? That's on Monday, November the 13th.

- ☐ 1週間おきに診察を受けに来てください。
  I want you to come see me every other week.

- ☐ 2週間後に診察を受けていただく必要があります。
  You need to come back to see me in two weeks.

⇨ 医師の立場から「診察を受けに来る」と言うのは come (to) see me、患者の視点から「診察を受けに行く」と言うのは go (to) see a doctor です。ちなみに「診察を受ける」は see a doctor、visit a doctor、consult with a doctor の言い方もあります。「2週間後」のように先の日にちの場合には Monday, November the 13th. などのように、日付を付け加えます。

予約が必要ない場合

- ☐ 数日経っても治らないようでしたら、診察に来てください。
  If it doesn't clear up in a few days, I want you to come back in.

- ☐ それを試してみて、まだ具合が悪いようなら診察に来てください。
  Why don't you try that and get back to me if you're still uncomfortable?

- ☐ 気分がよくならないようなら、診察しに来てください。
  You should come see me again if you don't feel better.

⇨ 特に次の予約は入れないけれども、何かあったら診察に来てくださいというときは、come back in「戻って来る」、come see me「やって来る」などを使います。

患者の予定を確認する

- ☐ 今から1ケ月後の月曜日の午前9時ではいかがですか。
  How about 9am on Monday, one month from now?

⇨ How about 〜?「〜はいかがですか」を使って具体的な曜日を指定し、患者の予定を確認しています。

- ☐ 次の金曜の午前10時に来ていただけますか。
  Could you come at 10am next Friday?
- ☐ 月曜日か木曜日に診療予約を取っていただけます。
  You can make an appointment with me either on Monday or Thursday.
- ☐ 通常は月曜日は都合がつけられます。
  I'm usually available on Monday.
- ☐ 明日の朝9時半に来ていただきたいと思います。
  I'd like you to come tomorrow at 9:30 in the morning.
- ☐ 来週水曜日11時でご都合はつきますか。
  Could you make it at 11 o'clock next Wednesday?

予約を確定する

- ☐ 月曜日の午前9時に予約を取ります。
  I'll put you down for Monday at 9am.

⇨ put 〜 down で「〜の名前を書きとめる、予約を取る」という意味です。

受付で次の診察日の予約を取ってもらう場合

- [ ] 次の診察日の予約を取ってください。
  Please make an appointment for your next visit.
- [ ] 受付で予約を取ってください。
  Please make an appointment with the receptionist.
- [ ] 受付係が予約を手配します。
  The receptionist will set up an appointment for you.

⇨ 医師の端末から予約日を入力して予約を確定せず、受付で予約を取る病院の場合、このような表現が必要になります。

手術・入院の予約を入れる

- [ ] できるだけ早く手術の予約を入れたいと思います。
  I'd like to schedule you for surgery as soon as possible.

⇨ schedule for ～で「～を予定に入れる、～の予定を決める」という意味になります。

- [ ] 入院受付で入院の予約をしてください。
  Please make an appointment for hospitalization at the admitting office.
- [ ] 手続きに必要な書類をお渡ししますが、それを下の階に持って行き、受付で処置の予約を入れていただく必要があります。
  I'll give you the paperwork, but you'll need to take it downstairs and schedule the procedure at one of the reception windows.

  ▶ paperwork：（手続きに必要な）書類

手術・入院の必要がない場合

- [ ] 手術の必要はないでしょう。
  You will not need to have surgery.
- [ ] 今のところ入院する必要はないと思います。何か特別な問題が見つかった場合には、入院していただくかもしれませんが。
  As of now, I don't think you have to stay overnight. If we find something especially troubling, we may want to admit you.

  ▶ admit：～を入院させる

3 次の予約を入れる

会話例 1

Dr. It's important to finish the entire course of antibiotics. Can you come back to see me two weeks from now? On Monday, the 27th.
大切なのは抗生物質投与の全過程を終えることです。2週間後に次の診察を受けに来ていただけますか。27日の月曜日です。

Pt. Actually, I'm not available that day. Would it be okay to come in on the following Wednesday morning?
実は、その日は都合がつきません。水曜の午前中ではいかがでしょうか。

Dr. Fine. I'll put you down for Wednesday, the 29th at 10 o'clock.
結構です。29日水曜日の10時に予約を入れます。

会話例 2

Dr. We can schedule your surgery for the 15th. You'll need to spend at least two weeks in the hospital.
手術を15日に入れることができます。あなたには少なくとも2週間入院していただく必要があります。

Pt. This is unbelievable. I'll have to miss a lot of work. I read about this surgery online in the US and even when they open people up like you're talking about, they let them go home that week.
これは信じられません。私は何日も仕事を休まねばなりません。アメリカで、ネットでこの手術について読みましたが、先生がおっしゃっている開腹手術を行っても、1週間で退院させています。

Dr. The Japanese system is different than what you're used to. Please understand that there are a lot of possible postsurgical complications.
日本のシステムはあなたが今まで受けてきたものとは異なります。この手術には数多くの術後合併症があることをご理解ください。

Pt. All right. I'll arrange to take time off for the surgery.
わかりました。手術のために休みをとります。

▶ postsurgical complication：術後合併症

Chapter 6 - 手術・入院

1 必要性・注意事項を説明する

手術や入院が必要な患者に対しては、その必要性を説明して理解してもらうことが大切です。

入院の必要性を伝える

☐ 腎臓病の処置が必要です。直ちに入院していただきたいと思います。
We need to deal with your kidney issues. I'd like to admit you right away.

⇨ 入院が必要となる理由を述べた上で、入院を促します。admit you は「あなたを入院させる」という意味です。「入院が必要です」は You need to be admitted to the hospital. や You need to be hospitalized. を使うこともできます。

☐ 精密検査を行いたいので、数日間入院していただきたいと思います。
I want to run more detailed tests, so I'd like you to check into the hospital for a few days.

⇨ check into the hospital は「入院する」の意味です。enter the hospital も使えます。その他、stay を使って表現することもできます。
stay overnight（1日入院する）
stay ～ days [weeks / months] in the hospital（～日［週／月］入院する）

手術の必要性を伝える

☐ 膀胱に明らかに石があります。そのうちの少なくとも1つは大型ですので、手術の予定を入れる必要があります。
There are definitely stones in your bladder. I see at least one of them is large, so I need to schedule you for surgery.

⇨ 必要性を患者によく説明し、納得してもらうことが大切です。surgery は、普通は数えられない名詞として使います。

☐ 他の治療からはわずかな痛みの軽減しか得られなかったので、椎間板ヘルニアの手術を検討すべきです。
You've had very little relief from other treatments, so we should consider surgery to remove the herniated disks.

- ☐ 腫瘍を取るために、手術が必要です。
  You need to have surgery to remove the tumor.
- ☐ 皮膚の腫瘍を取る手術が必要です。
  The growth on your skin needs to be surgically removed.
- ☐ より踏み込んだ治療を行いたいと思います。そのためもう一度手術を行いたいと思います。
  I'd like to be a little more aggressive with your treatment, so I'd like you to have another surgery.

⇨ 必要性を述べるには、should、need to ～などを用います。また、理由を述べるにはsoや目的を表すto不定詞などが使われます。

手術までの注意事項を伝える

- ☐ 同意書に署名をお願いします。
  We need you to sign the consent forms.
- ☐ 手術当日、署名された同意書をご持参ください。
  Please bring the signed consent form on the day of surgery.
- ☐ 手術前日の9時以降は飲食をしないようにしてください。
  Don't eat or drink anything after 9 o'clock the night before the surgery.
- ☐ その薬は手術の5日前に中止してください。
  I want you to stop that medication five days before surgery.
- ☐ 手術前日は、クリアリキッド（水やお茶、清涼飲料水など）以外は口にしないでください。
  You'll need to drink clear liquids only on the day before the surgery.
- ☐ アスピリンやその他の薬、あるいはここに掲載されているサプリメントは服用しないでください。
  Don't take any aspirin or any of the other drugs or supplements that are listed here.
- ☐ 手術前には真夜中以降は何も飲まないでください。日中は、澄んだスープやお茶の類は口にして結構です。
  Don't drink anything after midnight the day before surgery. During the day you can have clear soup, tea and that sort of thing.

会話例 1

Dr. We want to run some tests, so we'd like you to check into the hospital for a few days.
いくつか検査をしたいので、数日間入院していただきたいと思います。

Pt. What kind of tests?
どんな種類の検査ですか。

Dr. We'll start out with some simple neurological tests. We'll take some blood and we'll do an EEG.
簡単な神経学的検査から始めます。血液を採ってから、脳波の検査を行います。

Pt. Excuse me, but those sound like things I can do as an outpatient.
あのう、そうした検査は、通院でできる検査のように思えますが。

Dr. Ordinarily yes, but we want to see what your brainwaves are like in a variety of different situations—when you're awake, when you're asleep, and so forth.
普通はそうですが、私たちはあなたの脳波が、起きている時や眠っている時など、状況によってどうなるのかを調べたいのです。

▶ neurological test：神経学的検査　　EEG：脳波検査

会話例 2

Dr. I hear they even send people home the day of the surgery at some hospitals in the States. We like to keep patients at least overnight for observation, though.
米国では、手術後に患者さんに帰宅してもらう病院もあると聞いています。しかし当院では経過観察のため、患者さんには1泊していただいています。

Pt. I thought it was just the flu or food poisoning of some sort. I wasn't prepared for an operation.
私はただの風邪か何か食あたりだと思っていました。手術の準備はしていません。

Dr. I understand. Is there someone at home that can bring you a change of clothes or two and toiletries?
そうでしょうね。だれか2組ほどの着替えと洗面用具を持ってきてくれる方は家にいらっしゃいますか。

Pt. Probably ... I'll call my roommate.
たぶん…。ルームメートに電話します

● 会話例3

Dr. We need you to sign the consent forms. There's an English translation for you to look at so you know what you're signing.
　同意書に署名をお願いしたいと思います。英訳版がありますので、署名する内容についてご確認ください。

Pt. What's the purpose of all this?
　この同意書の目的はどういったことですか。

Dr. We try to follow the informed consent process. By signing, you acknowledge that you understand what's involved in your surgery based on both my explanation and the papers that I've given you.
　当院はインフォームドコンセントの遵守を心がけています。手術に関わることを、私からの説明とお渡した書面を元に、署名して承認していただくわけです。

Pt. All right.
　了解しました。

雑学
申込書・英語版フォーマット

　Chapter 1「総合受付」でも紹介しましたが、厚生労働省はホームページで、医療に関する「外国人向け多言語説明資料」を提供しています。
　「入院部門」や次章の「会計部門」についても日本語版と英語版をダウンロードできます。

【入院部門】
（1）入院申込書　　　　　　　（2）入院申込書（兼誓約書）
（3）入院歴の確認について　　（4）面会について
（5）感染予防について

【会計部門】
（1）高額療養費制度（限度額適用認定証）について
（2）出産一時金の直接支払制度の利用に関する合意確認書
（3）概算医療費　　　（4）医療費請求書　　　（5）医療費領収書

【手術・検査部門】
（1）～（3）麻酔問診票、麻酔に関する説明書・同意書
（4）～（5）輸血療法に関する説明書・同意書
（6）手術に関する説明書　　等々

Chapter 6 - 手術・入院

2 麻酔について質問・説明する

手術に必要不可欠なのが「麻酔」です。麻酔を行うには、事前に患者に対して十分に質問や説明を行う必要があります。

問題がないかを確認する

- ☐ 今まで麻酔によって異常が起きたことはありますか。
  Have you ever had problems with anesthesia?

- ☐ ご家族やご親せきに、麻酔薬で異常な反応を示した方はおられますか。
  Do you have any family members or relatives who have shown an abnormal reaction to anesthetics?"

  ▶ anesthesia：麻酔　　anesthetic：麻酔薬

- ☐ 血が止まりにくいですか
  Does your body have trouble stopping once you start bleeding?

- ☐ 入れ歯をしていますか。
  Do you have dentures?

- ☐ 何か食べ物や薬のアレルギーはありますか。
  Do you have any food or drug allergies?

- ☐ 当院で知っておくべき医療に影響を与えるような宗教的、文化的な習慣はありますか。
  Do you have any religious or cultural customs we need to know about that could affect your care?

⇨ 宗教や文化的な理由から「輸血（blood donation）」などが受け入れられない患者もいます。

リスクを説明する

- ☐ もちろん、私たちスタッフ一同は最善を尽くしますが、どんな処置にも合併症の危険性があるということをご理解ください。
  Of course all the staff will perform to give you the best care possible, but please understand that, as with every procedure, there is a risk of complications.

2 麻酔について質問・説明する

● 会話例 1　

Dr. Hello, I'm Dr. Tanaka. I'm going to be your anesthesiologist. I'd like to do a quick examination. I want to check your vitals, your weight and such ... Your medical history indicates you had surgery before, right?
こんにちは、医師の田中です。あなたの麻酔を担当します。簡単な診断をさせてください。あなたのバイタルサイン、体重などを測定しましょう。病歴を見ると、以前手術を受けられましたね。

Pt. Yes. I had my appendix out.
はい、盲腸を取りました。

Dr. Did you have any reaction to the anesthesia?
何か麻酔による副作用はありましたか。

Pt. No, that was fine.
いいえ、問題ありませんでした。

> ▶ anesthesiologist：麻酔医　　vitals：バイタルサイン（心拍数・呼吸数・血圧・体温）

● 会話例 2　

Dr. So, the surgeon already explained that you'll undergo general anesthesia ... is that right?
それで、もう外科の先生から、手術は全身麻酔で行うという説明は受けられましたね。

Pt. Yes, but I know general anesthesia can be risky ...
はい、でも全身麻酔はリスクがあると聞きますが。

Dr. When we know that an operation is going to take a long time, we use general anesthesia for various reasons. I'll give you a few ... you won't feel any pain, you won't be able to move around and your muscles will remain relaxed.
手術に時間がかかることがわかっているときは、私たちはさまざまな理由から全身麻酔を採択します。いくつか理由を挙げると、痛みを一切感じないこと、動けないこと、筋肉がリラックスした状態であることです。

Pt. Okay.
わかりました。

> ▶ general anesthesia：全身麻酔

Chapter 7 - 会計

1　会計窓口

診察が終わると、患者は会計窓口へ行きます。名前が呼ばれたら、精算窓口に行って支払いをしてもらいます。名前を呼ぶのではなくて、受付番号が掲示板に表示される病院もあります。診察後の手続きに関わる英語を見ていきましょう。

会計窓口で

☐ あなたのファイルを提出してください。
　Please turn in your folder.

☐ 席に座ってお名前が呼ばれるまでお待ちください。
　Please take a seat and wait until your name is called.

☐ お名前は精算窓口から呼ばれます。
　・Your name will be called from the cashier's desk [window].
　・They'll call your name from the casher's desk [window].

☐ お名前が呼ばれたら精算窓口で料金をお支払いください。
　Please pay the fees when you're called to the cashier desk's.

☐ こちらの待合室で順番までお待ちください。
　Please wait in this waiting room for your turn.

☐ 医療費の計算が終わりましたらお呼びします。
　You'll be called when your medical fees have been calculated.

☐ 支払いがお済みになると、領収書、次回の予約票、それから院内薬局、あるいは院外薬局で受け取れる処方箋が発行されます。
　After payment, you'll be issued a receipt, a next appointment slip and a prescription valid at the hospital pharmacy, as well as outside pharmacies.

● 会話例 1　　　　　　　　　　　　　　　　　　

R (Receptionist): May I have your folder? If this is your first visit this month, I also need to see your health insurance card.
　ファイルを提出していただけますか。今回が今月最初の来院でしたら、健康保険証もご提示

1 会計窓口

ください。

Pt. Here you are.
はい、これです。

R Please take a seat and wait until your name is called. They'll call your name from the cashier's desk.
席に着いてお名前が呼ばれるまでお待ちください。お名前は精算窓口から呼ばれます。

Pt. OK. About how long will I need to wait?
わかりました。どのくらい待つ必要がありますか。

R It usually takes 10 to 20 minutes to calculate the medical fees.
医療費を計算するのに10分から20分ほどかかります。

精算・支払い

☐ 本日の診察費は2000円になります。
The consultation fee for today comes to two thousand yen.

☐ 今日は2000円になります。
That will be two thousand yen.

☐ 本日の診察関係の費用は2000円になります。
The cost for today's services will be two thousand yen.

⇨ consultation fee の代わりにservicesを使うと、診察料だけでなく手術費や入院費などさまざまな明細を包括的に表すことができます。

☐ DC、VISA、MasterCard、JCBそれからAmerican Expressといったクレジットカードがお使いいただけます。
Payment by credit card such as DC, VISA, MasterCard, JCB and American Express will be accepted.

☐ 健康診断、予防接種、普通分娩、妊娠中絶、美容整形や視力測定などは、健康保険の対象になりません。
The public health insurance doesn't cover costs for regular check-ups, vaccination, normal childbearing, abortion, cosmetic surgery, or optometry.

Chapter 7 会計

クレジットが使えない場合

支払いにクレジットカードが使えるところが増えていますが、クレジットカードが使えない病院では次の表現を使います。

- ☐ クレジットカードは扱っておりません。現金でお支払いいただきたいと思います。
  We don't accept credit cards. We'd like you to pay in cash.

- ☐ 日本円でしかお支払いいただけません。
  We only accept Japanese yen.

- ☐ 1階のコンビニエンスストアの隣にATMがあります。そこで現金を引き出すことができます。
  There's an ATM on the 1st floor next to the convenience store. You can withdraw cash from there.

支払のあとで

支払いが終わると、患者は診察券（patient ID card）や処方箋（prescription）などを受け取ります。

- ☐ レシート、診察券、健康保険証、そして処方箋を受け取ってください。
  Please take the receipt, your patient ID card, health insurance card, and the prescription.

- ☐ 月の最初の診察時には健康保険証を必ずお持ちください。
  Please be sure to bring your health insurance card for the first visit of each month.

- ☐ 1階の薬局に行って処方箋の薬を調合してもらってください。
  Please go to the Pharmacy on the 1st floor to have your prescription filled.

- ☐ 院外薬局でも薬を受け取ることができます。
  You can also pick up your medicine at a pharmacy outside the hospital.

- ☐ 今日は薬が出ませんので、これでお帰りになって結構です。
  You may leave now as you don't need any medicine today.

☐ 再度来られる際には、診察券を忘れずにお持ちください。
Please do not forget to bring your patient ID card when you revisit the hospital.

● 会話例 2

C (Cashier): You're paying for the visit yourself, correct? Here's the bill.
自費診療ですね。料金はこちらになります。

Pt. Can I pay in dollars?
ドルで支払うことはできますか。

C We only accept yen. There's a bank in front of the hospital entrance. You can change dollars into yen there.
日本円でしかお支払いいただけません。病院入口の向かいに銀行があります。ドルを円に両替できます。

Pt. Ah, thank you for your help.
ああ、どうもありがとう。

● 会話例 3

C Here's the bill.
料金はこちらになります。

Pt. Do you accept this credit card?
このカードは使えますか。

C Sure. Here are your receipt and medical certificate. Oh, and this is your prescription. Take good care.
もちろんです。こちらが領収書と診断書です。それから処方箋も出ています。どうぞお大事に。

Pt. Thank you.
ありがとう。

Chapter 8 - ER（救急治療室）

1　救急措置

救急治療室（ER）には毎日多くの緊急を要する患者が担ぎ込まれ、医師たちが対応に追われます。症状によっては一刻を争うケースもあります。ここでは簡潔で的確な表現が求められます。

救急措置を行う

☐ 脈が取れません。心肺機能蘇生、開始！
I'm not getting a pulse. Start CPR!
▶ CPR（cardiopulmonary resuscitation）：心肺停止の蘇生救急、心肺蘇生

☐ 彼女（患者）を診察台に運びましょう。
Let's get her on the examination table.

☐ 彼（患者）を第一診察室に運びましょう。
Let's get him into Exam Room 1.

☐ バイタルサインはどんな具合ですか。
How are his vitals?

☐ GCSの数値はいくつですか。
What was her GCS score?

▶ **vitals**：バイタルサイン（vital signs）の略称。「生命の兆候」とも訳され、多くの場合、脈拍［心拍数］・呼吸（数）・血圧・体温の４つを指します。

GCS = Glasgow Coma Scale：グラスゴー・コーマ・スケール（グラスゴー昏睡尺度）＊開眼機能（Eye opening）「E」、言語機能（Verbal response）「V」、運動機能（Motor response）「M」の３分野に分けて記録し、意識状態を簡潔かつ的確に記録できます。記述は、「E_点、V_点、M_点、合計_点」と表現され、正常は15点満点で深昏睡は3点。点数は小さいほど重症です。
Severe（重度）：GCS 3-8　　Moderate（中度）：GCS 9-12　　Mild（軽度）：GCS 13-15
なお、日本では、簡便なJapan Coma Scaleジャパン・コーマ・スケール（JCS）が広く用いられています。

☐ 点滴をします。
・**We will put you on an IV drip.**
・**We will put you on a drip.**

⇨ 「点滴」はan intravenous dripと言いますが、IntraVenous（静脈内の）を略してan IV drip、あるいはdripだけでもよく用いられます。put you onの他に、give youも用いられます。

1 救急措置

会話例 1

Dr.1 He's badly burned.
患者はひどい火傷を負っています。

Dr.2 How are his vitals?
バイタルサインはどんな具合ですか。

Dr.1 I'm not getting a pulse. Start CPR!
脈が取れません。心肺機能蘇生、開始！

会話例 2

P.M. (Patient's mother): My daughter hit her head this morning when she fell outside. There wasn't much blood, but she started vomiting for apparently no reason about two hours ago.
娘は外で転んで、今朝頭を打ったんです。血はあまり出ませんでしたが、2時間前にはっきりした理由もなく吐き始めました。

Dr. Let's get her on the examination table. I want to run a few tests and then maybe do a scan.
彼女を診察台に運びましょう。数件の検査をして、その後、スキャンをしたいと思います。

会話例 3

P.W. (Patient's wife): My husband hit his head and lost consciousness.
夫は頭を打って意識を失ったんです。

Dr.1 Sir, sir, do you know where you are?
もしもし、どこにいらっしゃるかわかりますか。

Pt. Hhh-hospital.
びょ、病院です。

Dr.2 Let's get him into Exam Room 1.
患者さんを第一診察室に運びましょう。

● 会話例 4

Dr.1 Excuse me, Dr. Thomas, could I get your opinion on this patient? She's nine years old. She hit her head earlier today and has been vomiting.

トーマス先生、すみません、この患者さんについての先生の意見をお聞かせいただけますか。患者さんは9歳で、今朝早くに頭を打ち、嘔吐エピソードが続いています。

Dr.2 What was her GCS score?

GCS（グラスゴー昏睡尺度）の数値はいくつですか。

Dr.1 I put it at about 12.

だいたい12とみなしています。

Dr.2 Hmm ... that's just beyond the mild level, so it's moderate. I don't like to order unnecessary tests, but I think we should do a scan to be on the safe side.

ええと、その数値だと中度を少し超えただけですから、軽度と言えます。私は不必要な検査を指示したくないのですが、大事をとってスキャンを行うべきだと思います。

● 会話例 5

N We'd like to put you on a drip. Let's have you lie down over here.

点滴をしたいと思います。ここに横になってください。

Pt. Do you prefer the right arm or the left?

右腕がいいですか、左腕がいいですか。

N Either is fine.

どちらの腕でも結構です。

表現のポイント

嘔吐（吐く）に関する表現

★ **Written, Formal**（正式な文書表現）
　…emetic episode　嘔吐エピソード（病状の発現）

★ **Neutral**（書き言葉にも話し言葉にも使える）
　…vomit, throw up

★ **Spoken**（話し言葉）…puke, upchuck

★ **Very Casual**（非常にカジュアルな言葉）…hurl, barf

救急措置後に家族に説明する

☐ 患者さんは安定しています。
　We've stabilized him.

☐ すでに患者さんに緩和な鎮痛剤を投与してあります。
　We've already given him a mild sedative.

▶ stabilize：〜を安定させる　　mild sedative：緩和な鎮静薬

● 会話例 6

Dr. Your husband has severe burns. He was having some trouble breathing, but we've stabilized him. We need to admit him for further treatment.
ご主人は重度の火傷です。呼吸に問題がありましたが、安定しています。さらに治療をしたいので、入院していただきます。

P.W. (Patient's wife): What should I do?
私は何をしたらいいでしょうか。

Dr. You need to go downstairs to Window 1 where it says, "Hospital Admittance," and take care of all the paperwork.
下の階の「入院」と書かれた1番窓口に行って、すべての事務書類に対応してください。

● 会話例 7

Dr. We've given him something for the fever. I'd like you to apply cool compresses to his forehead or other pulse points to help bring it down further.
患者さんには熱の薬を飲んでいただきました。もっと熱を下げるために、おでこや脈を打っている部分に冷たい湿布をあてがってください。

P.M. (Patient's mother): How often?
どのくらいの頻度ですか。

Dr. At least five or six times a day.
少なくとも1日に5、6回お願いします。

▶ cool compress：冷湿布
　pulse points：パルスポイント（手首や耳の後ろなど脈を感じるところ、身体の中で体温の高い部分）

Chapter 8 · ER (救急治療室)

雑学
手術を表す用語について

接尾辞 -ectomy

「〜切除術」の意味を持ち、体の一部を切除・摘出する手術に多く用いられています。
  例) spleen (脾臓) + -ecotomy = splenectomy (脾臓摘出術)
      appendix (虫垂) + -ectomy = appendectomy (虫垂切除)
      または appendicectomy、appendisectomy
      gastr (entire stomach) (胃全部) + -ectomy = gastrectomy (胃切除)
      hemorrhoids (痔) + -ectomy = hemorrhoidectomy (痔核切除)
全部ではなく部分的な切除術を示すものもあります。
  例) vas deferens (精管) + -ectomy = vasectomy (精管切除)
  また新語である lumpectomy (腫瘍摘出手術) は breast (乳房) から lump (しこり) を除去する手術です。乳房全体を取り除く手術は mastectomy (乳房切除術) と呼ばれます。

接尾辞 -otomy

「〜切開術」の意味を持ちます。
  例) trachea (気管) + -otomy = tracheotomy (気管切開術)
      perineum (会陰) + -otomy = episiotomy、perineotomy (会陰切開術)

米国で最も一般的な手術10 (アルファベット順)

1.	Angioplasty; atherectomy	血管形成
2.	Broken bone repair	骨折治療
3.	C-section delivery	帝王切開による出産
4.	Cataract removal	白内障手術
5.	Circumcision	陰茎切除
6.	Gallbladder removal (cholecystectomy)	胆嚢摘出術
7.	Heart bypass surgery (coronary artery bypass graft)	心臓バイパス手術 (冠動脈バイパス移植)
8.	Hysterectomy	子宮摘出術
9.	Joint replacement (knee and hip replacements)	関節置換術 (膝および股関節置換手術)
10.	Stent procedure	ステント術

PART 2 応用編

応用編では、
各診療科別に使えるフレーズを紹介します。
実際の診察場面の会話と
診療科で使えるフレーズを、
専門的な表現や用語の説明を交えて
解説しています。

Chapter 1 - 神経内科

1 神経痛 ●●● Nerve Pain

神経内科のDr. Adachiの診察室です。患者は数年前に米国で坐骨神経痛と診断されており、慢性的な痛みに悩まされています。日本で診断を受けるのは今日が初めてなのですが…。 CD2-01

Dr. All right, it says here that you've been suffering from chronic pain. Could you describe it for me?

Pt. I get a pins and needles feeling in my leg on and off. Otherwise, it's kind of numb. Sometimes my leg just aches and gets kind of hot. When the pain medicine wears off, it is a dull ache that is a bit difficult to describe. I was diagnosed with a pinched nerve and sciatica a few years ago.

Dr. Apparently you still have some nerve entrapment going on. The medication you've been taking that you got in the U.S. is usually only prescribed for cancer patients in Japan.

Pt. Oh…

Dr. So, I'm going to prescribe something a bit milder that should have a similar effect on the pain. It's a combination drug that includes two types of painkillers. Why don't we give it a month and see how you do?

Pt. All right. Thank you.

Dr. I'm also prescribing ten days of stomach medicine. Some people have a reaction to the drug that includes nausea or stomach issues, so this is just a precaution.

語句・表現

chronic pain：慢性痛、慢性の痛み
pins and needles：(脚などが)チクチク何かに刺されているような感覚
numb：しびれた、まひした
pinched nerve：圧迫による神経痛
sciatica：坐骨神経痛
nerve entrapment：神経絞扼（末梢神経が隣接組織から障害・炎症を受けた状態）
painkiller：鎮痛剤
reaction：反応、副作用
nausea：吐き気
precaution：予防策、予防措置

1 神経痛 ●●● Nerve Pain

訳

D：わかりました。ここに、あなたは慢性的な痛みに悩まされていると書かれています。症状を説明していただけますか。

P：足に断続的にチクチク何かに刺されているような感じがあります。それとしびれた感じもあります。足がただ痛くて熱を帯びていることもあります。鎮痛剤の効果が薄れてくると、少し説明が難しいのですが、鈍い痛みがあります。数年前に圧迫による神経痛および坐骨神経痛と診断されました。

D：明らかにあなたは、今でも神経絞扼の状態にあります。あなたが米国で入手し服用されている薬は、通常日本ではがんの患者さんの痛みにのみ処方されています。

P：まあ！

D：ですから、痛みに対して同様の効果のある、もう少し穏やかなものを処方します。これは2種類の鎮痛剤を含んだ配合剤です。1ヶ月分処方しますから、様子を見ましょう。

P：わかりました。ありがとうございます。

D：10日分の胃薬も処方します。この薬に対する作用として吐き気や胃のトラブルを起こす人がいますので、これは単に予防措置です。

表現のポイント

患者は太字の語以外はいずれも簡単な英単語を組み合わせることで症状を具体的に説明しています。

★ I get a **pin and needles** feeling in my leg on and off.
　足が断続的にチクチク何かに刺されているような感じがあります。

★ Otherwise, it's kind of **numb**.
　それとしびれた感じもあります。

★ Sometimes my leg just aches and gets kind of hot.
　足がただ痛くて熱を帯びていることもあります。

★ When the pain medicine wears off, it is a dull ache that is a bit difficult to describe.
　鎮痛剤の効果が薄れてくると、少し説明が難しいのですが、鈍い痛みがあります。
　*wear off（痛みや効果が）徐々に消えていく

★ I was diagnosed with a **pinched nerve** and **sciatica** few years ago.
　数年前に圧迫による神経痛および坐骨神経痛と診断されました。
　*be diagnosed with 〜　〜と診断される

Chapter 1 - 神経内科

●●● 神経内科　使える表現

症状をたずねる

☐ **Dr.** 症状を説明していただけますか。
✪ Could you describe it for me?
Pt. 足に断続的にチクチク何かに刺されているような感じがあります。
✪ I get a pins and needles feeling in my leg on and off.

☐ **Dr.** うずくような痛みに最初に気づいたのはいつですか。
When did you first notice the tingling?
Pt. 先週、バスケットボールをしてから始まりました。
It started after I played basketball last week.
▶ tingling：うずくような痛み

☐ **Dr.** 足にしびれや痛みを感じたことはありますか。
Have you felt any numbness or pain in your legs?
Pt. はい。特に左足にしびれを感じます。
Yes. I feel some numbness, especially in my left leg.
▶ numbness：しびれ

☐ **Dr.** 常に痛みがあるとおっしゃいましたね。
Would you say that you're in constant pain?
Pt. いいえ、現れたり消えたりすると申しました。
No, I'd say it comes and goes.
▶ be in constant pain：常に痛みがある
　come and go：現れたり消えたりする

☐ **Dr.** 痛みについてお話ください。
Tell me about the pain.
Pt. 断続的に痛みます。夜の方が楽です。
It hurts on and off. It's better at night.
▶ on and off：断続的に

☐ **Dr.** 痛みについてもっと詳しくお聞きしたいと思います。
I'd like to hear more details about your pain.
Pt. 腕が痛くて、熱を帯びています。鎮痛剤の効果が薄れると、上半身全体が歯痛のような感じになります。
My arm aches and gets kind of hot. When the pain medicine wears off, it feels like an entire upper body toothache.

1 神経痛 ●●● Nerve Pain

診断

□ あなたは、今でも神経絞扼の状態にあります。

❋ You still have some nerve entrapment going on.

□ 脊髄狭窄症の兆候もあります。

There are also signs of spinal stenosis.
> spinal stenosis：脊髄管狭窄症

□ この検査に対する反応からすると、あなたは坐骨神経痛でしょう。

Based on your reactions to this test, I believe you have sciatica.

処置・処方

□ 痛みに対して同様の効果のある、もう少し穏やかなものを処方します。

❋ I'm going to prescribe something a bit milder that should have a similar effect on the pain.

□ 1ヶ月分処方しますから、様子を見ましょう。

❋ Why don't we give it a month and see how you do?

□ 痛みやしびれを抑えるかどうか見るために、あなたに理学療法を試していただきたいと思います。

I'd like you to try physical therapy to see if that helps with the pain and numbness.

□ コーチゾン注射をお勧めします。短時間で作用する麻酔剤とステロイドが組み合わさったものです。神経への抗炎症作用があるので、痛みを和らげ、神経圧迫そのものを軽減するはずです。

I recommend a cortisone injection, which combine steroids with a short-acting anesthetic. There's an anti-inflammatory effect and this will decrease the pressure on the nerve itself.
> cortisone：コーチゾン（リウマチの治療用ホルモン）
> anesthetic：麻酔薬、麻酔剤
> anti-inflammatory effect：抗炎症作用
> pressure on the nerve：神経圧迫

Chapter 1 - 神経内科

2　頭痛 ●●● Headache

頭痛を引き起こす原因や症状はさまざまです。Dr. Adachiはじっくり検査をし、結論を急がないように勧めています。

Dr. So, according to your chart, you've been suffering from incessant headaches?

Pt. That's right. I saw an ENT and he couldn't find anything wrong with my sinuses, so he sent me to you.

Dr. Could you describe it for me?

Pt. The pain is strongest around my eyes and face. In addition to a constant ache, I feel a lot of pressure. I saw my dentist before that and the pain is not coming from my teeth, either.

Dr. Does it hurt worse when you lie down or bend?

Pt. I don't think so.

Dr. You may actually have some sort of infection that's causing the headaches. I'd like to rule out… meningitis, for example. I can order a full neurological work-up and we can do a CSF, cerebrospinal fluid analysis, but I'd like to start with some simple bloodwork. Actually, let's get a urine sample, as well.

Pt. Wow, this sounds serious.

Dr. Let's not jump to any conclusions yet. You've answered all the questions on our usual medical history questionnaire, but I'd like to have you sit down with my PA and give her a very detailed medical history. I'd also like you to tell her if you've had any insect bites or anything else out of the ordinary in the past few months.

語句・表現

incessant：絶え間ない（non-stopのフォーマル表現、恒常的な痛みに用いられる）
ENT (ear nose throat)：耳鼻咽喉科
sinuses：洞、副鼻腔
infection：感染症
rule out ～：～を除外する、排除する
meningitis：髄膜炎
neurological：神経学的な

2 頭痛 ●●● Headache

訳

D：それでカルテによると、あなたは絶えず頭痛に悩まされているのですね。

P：そうなんです。私は耳鼻咽喉科を受診しましたが、副鼻腔には何も問題は見つかりませんでした。それで先生に診てもらうようにと言われたのです。

D：症状を説明していただけますか。

P：痛みは目と顔の周辺が最もひどいです。絶えず痛むだけでなく、強い圧迫感があります。それ以前には歯科を受診しましたが、痛みは歯が原因でもなさそうです。

D：横になったり屈んだりすると痛みはひどくなりますか。

P：それはないと思います。

D：実際は、あなたは何らかの感染症にかかっていて、それが頭痛を起こしていると思われます。例えば…髄膜炎でないことを確認したいと思います。神経学的な精密検査全般や、脳脊髄液の分析もできますが、簡単な血液検査から始めたいと思います。実際に、尿検査もしておきましょう。

P：わあ、重症のようですね。

D：まだ、結論を出すのは早計です。当院で通常行う病歴の問診票にはすべて答えていただいていますが、PA（医療助手）にあなたの病歴を詳しく伝えてください。過去数ヶ月の間に、虫に刺されたり、いつもとは違ったことがあればそれも話していただきたいと思います。

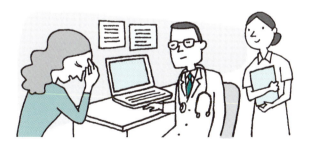

---

work-up：（問診・レントゲン検査などを含む）精密検査
CSF (cerebrospinal fluid)：脳脊髄液
bloodwork (=blood test)：血液検査
urine sample：尿サンプル
PA (physician assistant)：医師助手

Chapter 1 · 神経内科

神経内科　使える表現

症状をたずねる

- **Dr.** 症状を説明していただけますか。
  Could you describe it for me?
  Pt. 痛みは目と顔の周辺が最もひどいです。絶えず痛むだけでなく、強い圧迫感があります。
  ❀ The pain is strongest around my eyes and face. In addition to a constant ache, I feel a lot of pressure.

- **Dr.** どうなさいましたか。
  What seems to be the trouble?
  Pt. ひどい頭痛が続いています。
  I keep getting terrible headaches.

- **Pt.** 1週間、首が痛くて死にそうです。
  My neck has been killing me for a week.
  Dr. 拝見しましょう。
  Let's have a look.

- 横になったり屈んだりすると痛みはひどくなりますか。
  ❀ Does it hurt worse when you lie down or bend?

- **Pt.** こめかみがずきずきします。
  My temples are throbbing.
  Dr. どのくらい続いていますか。
  How long has this been going on?
  ▶ temple：こめかみ　　throbbing：ずきずきする

- **Pt.** もう1週間ずきずきする頭痛があります。
  I've had a pounding [throbbing] headache for a week now.
  Dr. 症状を確認するためいくつか検査を行いましょう。
  Let's run some tests to see what's going on.
  ▶ pounding：ずきずきする

診断

- あなたは一般的な緊張性頭痛だと思います。
  I believe you are having simple tension headaches.
  ▶ tension headache：緊張性[型]頭痛

2 頭痛 ●●● Headache

- [ ] あなたの病状は偏頭痛のように思われます。

  Your problem sounds like migraine headaches.
  - migraine headache：偏頭痛

- [ ] 何らかの感染症にかかっていて、それが頭痛を起こしていると思われます。

  You may have some sort of infection that's causing the headaches.

- [ ] 明らかにあなたの鼻腔に問題があり、それが頭痛を引き起こしています。

  There is definitely a problem with your sinuses that's causing the headache.

治療・助言

- [ ] 気化器か加湿器を入手していただきたいと思います。部屋の空気の湿気を保つ必要があります。

  I'd like you to get a vaporizer or humidifier. You need to keep the air in your room moist.
  - vaporizer：気化器、噴霧器　　humidifier：加湿器

- [ ] まずやっていただきたいのは、明るい光、アルコール、喫煙、大きな音といった、刺激性のものをなくすことです。

  The first thing you need to do is eliminate irritants such as bright lights, alcohol, smoke and loud noise.
  - irritant：いらいらさせるもの、刺激性のもの

- [ ] 休息できる涼しくて暗い場所を確保するようお勧めします。

  I recommend that you find a cool dark place to rest.

- [ ] 額に湿布を貼り、目を閉じてください。続いて、ゆっくり深く息を吸うリラクセーション療法を行ってください。

  Place a cool compress on your forehead and then close your eyes. Follow up with relaxation techniques taking slow, deep breaths.
  - compress：湿布　　take slow, deep breaths：ゆっくり深く息を吸う

Chapter 2 - 消化器内科

1　潰瘍性大腸炎　●●●　UC (Ulcerative Colitis)

消化器内科のDr. Babaは潰瘍性大腸炎の状態にある患者を診察しています。以前から下痢症状に苦しんでいたようです。

Dr. I understand you're having some digestive issues. Could you walk me through it?

Pt. The diarrhea is the main problem. I never know when I'm going to have an attack.

Dr. Have you noticed any blood in your stool?

Pt. I've seen a small amount of blood a few times, but not recently. The other thing is that I often have to go all of a sudden, I just barely make it to the toilet.

Dr. Some diseases do have that symptom of urgency.

Pt. Well, the other strange thing is that other times I feel like I have to go and I rush to the bathroom and then I don't have to do anything after all.

Dr. I suspect that this may be some sort of inflammatory bowel disease — I'm guessing we may be looking at ulcerative colitis. You're in your late twenties, right? Have you lost any weight recently?

Pt. As a matter of fact, yes. I'm two or three kilos lighter than I was two months ago.

Dr. Why didn't you come in sooner?

Pt. I felt a little better for a while and then it started all over again.

Dr. Well, let's start out with a couple of simple tests. I'd like to do some bloodwork and give you a kit. You'll need to collect a stool sample and bring it back for us to analyze.

1 潰瘍性大腸炎　●●● UC

訳

D：消化機能に問題があるようですね。それを詳しく説明していただけますか。

P：主な問題は下痢です。いつ起こるかまったくわかりません。

D：便に血が混じったことはありますか。

P：数回少量の血が出たことがありますが、最近はありません。他の問題としては突然便意をもよおし、かろうじてトイレに間に合うということがよくあります。

D：そうした切迫した症状をともなう病気もあるんです。

P：そうですね、それに奇妙なことには便意をもよおし、トイレに駆け込むのですが結局何も出ないことがあるんです。

D：これは炎症性腸疾患の類ではないかと思います。潰瘍性大腸炎かもしれないと推察しています。あなたは20台後半ですよね。最近体重は減りましたか。

P：実はそうなんです。2ヶ月前と比べると2、3kg減っています。

D：なぜもっと早く受診に来なかったのですか。

P：しばらく少しよくなっているように感じて、その後再び始まりました。

D：では、2、3の簡単な検査を始めましょう。いくつか血液検査を行いますので、検査キットをお渡します。分析のため便のサンプルを採取して、提出してください。

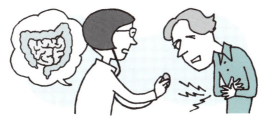

語句・表現

ulcerative colitis (UC)：潰瘍性大腸炎
digestive：消化の
walk ～ through it：そのことを～に詳しく説明する
diarrhea：下痢

attack：発作、発病
stool：便、排泄物
inflammatory bowel disease：炎症性大腸疾患

消化器内科　使える表現

症状をたずねる

☐ 便に血が混じったことはありますか。
❋ Have you noticed any blood in your stool?

☐ **Dr.** 出血の量はどのくらいですか。
How much blood is there?
Pt. 少量が2、3回ありました。
There was a small amount two or three times.

☐ 下痢の原因で思いあたることはありますか。
Do you have any idea what triggers these bouts of diarrhea?

☐ 1日に何回下痢をしますか。
How many times a day do you have diarrhea?

☐ 最近体重は減りましたか。
❋ Have you lost any weight recently?

検査

☐ いくつか血液検査を行いますので、検査キットをお渡しします。
❋ I'd like to do some bloodwork and give you a kit.

☐ 分析のため便のサンプルを採取して、提出してください。
❋ You'll need to collect a stool sample and bring it back for us to analyze.

☐ 貧血や感染を調べるための血液検査を2、3行い、便のサンプルもとりたいと思います。
I want to run a few blood tests to check for anemia or infection and then I'd also like to get a stool sample.
▶ anemia：貧血

☐ 炎症している正確な場所も突き止めたいので、来月に大腸内視鏡検査の予約を入れましょう。
I'd also like to locate the exact area of inflammation, so let's schedule you for a colonoscopy in the next month.
▶ inflammation：炎症　　colonoscopy：大腸内視鏡検査

診断・処方

☐ あなたは潰瘍性大腸炎ではないかと推測しています。

🌀 I'm guessing we may be looking at ulcerative colitis.

☐ あなたは潰瘍性大腸炎ではないかと思います。

We think you might have ulcerative colitis.

☐ 大腸内視鏡検査によると、あらゆることが潰瘍性大腸炎を示しています。

Based on your colonoscopy, everything points to UC.

☐ 大便サンプルに白血球が見られましたが、これは潰瘍性大腸炎のかなり大きな裏付けとなります。

There were white blood cells in your stool sample, which pretty much confirms the diagnosis of ulcerative colitis.
▶ white blood cell：白血球

☐ この新しい薬がどう作用するか見たいので、2、3週間後にまた受診してください。

I'd like to see you again in two to three weeks to see how you're doing on this new medication.

日常生活のアドバイス

☐ 投薬に加えて、日常の飲食物に注意していただきたいと思います。

In addition to the medication, I'd like you to watch your diet.

☐ 何か発症を起こす食材があったら、それを摂取するのを制限するか避けてください。

If you see that something triggers an attack, you want to limit or avoid it.

☐ 潰瘍性大腸炎の患者さんの多くは、乳製品が消化しにくいと感じています。少量の食事を摂ることも心がけてください。

Many people with UC find dairy foods difficult to digest. You may also want to consider eating small meals.

☐ ストレスの度合いに気をつけてください。

Keep an eye on your stress levels.

☐ 適度な運動もまた、症状を落ち着かせるのに効果があります。

Moderate exercise is good for calming things down.

Chapter 2 - 消化器内科

2 / 胃潰瘍 ●●● Ulcers

消化器内科のDr. Babaの患者は胃の痛みやむかつきを訴えています。
胃潰瘍の疑いがあるようです。

Dr. You say you've been having stomach pain? Could you show me exactly where?

Pt. Here.

Dr. That's kind of high up… Could you describe the pain?

Pt. Yeah, it's kind of a burning pain.

Dr. Do you feel nauseated?

Pt. Yes. I feel sick to my stomach a lot. One or two times, I've actually vomited. Once was after I'd eaten, so all my food came up, and the other time it was mostly bile.

Dr. Is there any history of ulcers in your family?

Pt. Actually, my father had ulcers.

Dr. Would you say you drink alcohol regularly?

Pt. I guess I have something to drink a few times a week.

Dr. Do you take aspirin or ibuprofen regularly?

Pt. I started taking an aspirin a day two years ago.

Dr. I suspect we may be dealing with ulcers here. Let's start you on an acid-blocking medication and see what happens with that. I'd like to see you again in three or four weeks to reassess the situation. I also suggest that you lay off the aspirin for the time being. You should also limit your dairy intake.

Pt. No, problem. I haven't been eating much dairy since I came to Japan.

2 胃潰瘍 ●●● Ulcers

訳

D：胃の痛みがあるとのことですね。正確にどこの部分か教えていただけますか。

P：ここです。

D：上の方ですね。痛みを説明していただけますか。

P：ええ、焼けるような痛みです。

D：吐き気はありますか。

P：はい。胃がとてもむかむかしています。実際に、1、2度吐きました。1度目は食後で、食べたものをすべて吐きましたし、別の時はほとんどが胆汁でした。

D：ご家族に胃潰瘍の病歴はありますか。

P：実は、父が胃潰瘍でした。

D：日常的にお酒を飲まれますか。

P：週に数回、何か飲むと思います。

D：定期的にアスピリンやイブプロフェンを服用されていますか。

P：2年前に1日1錠のアスピリンを服用し始めました。

D：胃潰瘍の治療をすることになるのではと思います。制酸薬から始めて、それでどうなるか様子を見ましょう。3、4週間後に再診していただき、症状を見直したいと思います。当分の間、アスピリンも止めることもお勧めします。乳製品の摂取も制限するべきです。

P：問題ありません。日本に来てからはあまり乳製品は摂っていません。

語句・表現

burning pain：焼けるような痛み、灼熱痛
feel sick to one's stomach：吐き気がする、胃がむかむかする
bile：胆汁
ibuprofen：イブプロフェン（非ステロイド系の解熱、鎮痛、抗炎症薬で、アスピリンより副作用が少ない）
take an aspirin a day：1日1錠のアスピリンを服用する
acid-blocking medication：制酸剤
reassess：〜を再評価する、見直す

消化器内科　使える表現

症状をたずねる

☐ 具体的にどこに腹痛があるか教えていただけますか。

Could you show me exactly where you've been having stomach pain?

☐ 吐き気はありますか。

❂ Do you feel nauseated?

☐ 吐きましたか。

Have you been vomiting?

☐ 吐いたものの様子を教えていただけますか。

Could I ask you to describe the appearance of the vomit?

☐ 食後は食べ物が胃にもたれますか。

Does food sit heavy in your stomach after you eat?

☐ ご家族に胃潰瘍の病歴はありますか。

❂ Is there any history of ulcers in your family?

処方・投薬への注意

☐ 制酸薬から始めて、それでどうなるか様子を見ましょう。

❂ Let's start you on an acid-blocking medication and see what happens with that.

☐ これをしばらく服用していただき、経過を観察します。

We are going to have you take this for a while and monitor your progress.

☐ この薬は、長期間服用しなければならないようなものではありませんが、あなたがおっしゃっている多くの症状にとても効果的です。

This isn't something you should take over a long period of time, but it can be very effective for many of the symptoms you've reported.

2 胃潰瘍 ●●● Ulcers

- [ ] この薬は胃潰瘍の治療と治癒の助けとなります。
  This medicine helps treat and heal the ulcers.

- [ ] 定期的にアスピリンやイブプロフェンを服用されていますか。
  Do you take aspirin or ibuprofen regularly?

- [ ] 当分の間、アスピリンも止めることをお勧めします。
  I'd like you to stop your daily aspirin regime for the time being.

- [ ] 乳製品の摂取も制限するべきです。
  You should also limit your dairy intake.

- [ ] 副作用の可能性がありますので、何か問題があれば直ちに私に連絡してください。
  There can be side effects, so I want you to let me know immediately if you have any issues.

- [ ] 呼吸に問題が出始めたら直ちに服用を止め、病院の診察を受けてください。
  If you start having trouble breathing, you need to stop taking the drug immediately and get to a hospital.

治療・手術

- [ ] **Pt.** 入院しなければなりませんか。
  Will I have to stay overnight?
  Dr. たぶんしなくてよいでしょう。ひどい出血といった、何か特別な問題が見つかった場合には、入院をお願いするかもしれませんが。
  Probably not. If they find something especially troubling, like severe bleeding, though, they may want to admit you.

- [ ] 私たちは潰瘍の手術は避けるようにしているのですが、あなたの症例では、外科医が加わり、穿孔を縫合しなければなりません。
  We try to avoid surgery with ulcers, but in your case, a surgeon has to go in and sew up the perforation.
  ▶ perforation：穿孔

- [ ] 内視鏡検査中にレーザーを使って出血を止めることができたので、手術の必要はないでしょう。
  We were able to stop the bleeding using a laser during the endoscopy, so you will not need to have surgery.

Chapter 3 - 腎臓内科

1　腎臓病 ... Kidney Failure

腎臓内科のDr. Chibaは腎臓病ということで紹介された若い患者を診察しています。

Dr. I'm a nephrologist. Dr. Ito wanted me to take a look at you and go over the results of your blood tests. I understand that in addition to the decreased urine output, you're experiencing fatigue?

Pt. Yes, I'm constantly tired. I also find myself horribly bloated because I don't seem to be able to urinate normally.

Dr. Fluid retention can be a sign of kidney disease. Are there any other symptoms?

Pt. I'm nauseous a lot of the time, as well.

Dr. I'm looking at the results of the blood tests and your GFR is 68. That's rather low in someone your age.

Pt. I'm not sure I understand what GFR is.

Dr. It stands for glomerular filtration rate, which is actually how much blood passes through the glomeruli in your kidneys per minute. Filtering waste from the blood is one of the main purposes of the kidneys, so the GFR test lets us know how well this is being done. If you were much older, I'd be a little less concerned, but you're young and you have several of the symptoms we see when the kidneys are not quite performing up to snuff. For all of these reasons, I want to run several more tests.

語句・表現

nephrologist：腎臓専門医
urine output：尿排出量
bloated：むくんだ
fluid retention：水分貯留

GFR (glomerular filtration rate)：糸球体ろ過率
not up to snuff：満足のいく状態にない、基準に達していない

1 腎臓病 ●●● Kidney Failure

訳

D： 私は腎臓専門医です。伊藤先生からあなたを診察し、血液検査の結果を調べるよう依頼されました。尿排出量の低下に加えて、疲労感があるのですね。

P： はい。いつも疲労を感じます。正常に排尿できていないようなので、ひどくむくんでいることにも気がつきました。

D： 体内に水がたまるのは腎臓病の兆候と言えます。他には何か症状はありますか。

P： しょっちゅう吐き気もあります。

D： 血液検査の結果を見ていますが、GFR（糸球体ろ過率）が68あります。あなたの年齢の人からするとちょっと低すぎます。

P： GFRが何なのかよくわからないのですが。

D： GFRはglomerular filtration rateの略で、1分間にあなたの腎臓においてどれだけの量の血液が糸球体を通過するかを示します。腎臓の主な役割は、血液から老廃物をろ過することですから、GFRを検査することで、この機能がどの程度保たれているかを知ることができます。あなたがもっと年をとっていれば、あまり気にしないのですが、あなたは若いですし、腎臓が十分には機能していないときに見るようないくつかの症状を持っておられます。こうしたすべての理由から、あといくつかの検査を受けていただきたいと思います。

表現のポイント

腎臓疾患を見極める検査

★ 尿排出量検査　urine output measurements
　1日の尿排出量を検査する。
★ 尿検査　urinalysis
　腎不全（kidney failure）を示唆する異常を明らかにする。
★ 血液検査　blood tests
　尿素窒素（urea nitrogen）およびクレアチニン（creatinine）値の急激な上昇を明らかにする。
★ 画像検査　imaging tests
　超音波（ultrasound）やCT（computed tomography）を用いて検査する。
★ 腎生検　kidney biopsy
　針を用いて腎臓の細胞を検査用サンプルとして取り出して検査する。

腎臓内科　使える表現

症状をたずねる

☐ 今までに、何か腎臓病の問題はありましたか。

Have you ever had any issues with kidney disease before?

☐ 尿排出量の低下に加えて、疲労感があるのですね。

❁ I understand that in addition to the decreased urine output, you're experiencing fatigue?

☐ 足のむくみや尿の量の減少の他に何か症状はありますか。

Have you had other symptoms besides the swelling in your legs and decreased urine output?

診断

☐ 血液検査の結果を見ていますが、GFR（糸球体ろ過率）が68あります。あなたの年齢の人からするとちょっと低すぎます。

❁ I'm looking at the results of the blood tests and your GFR is 68. That's rather low in someone your age.

☐ これは腎不全に見られるような深刻な症状だとわかっていますので、すぐに精密検査をしたいと思います。

I know this is a serious symptom that may indicate renal failure, so I want to take a further look right away.
　▶ renal failure：腎不全

☐ 結論は急がないようにしましょう。血液と尿の検査を行い、今の状況を判断したいと思います。

Let's not jump to conclusions. I'd like to do some blood and urine tests and determine what's going on now.

☐ 腎不全ではないかと思いますが、あなたのように若くて健康な人は回復可能でしょう。

I suspect some sort of renal failure, but it can be reversible in someone young and healthy like you.
　▶ reversible：回復可能な

☐ あなたは週3回の透析が必要です。

You'll need to go for dialysis three times a week.
　▶ dialysis：透析

1 腎臓病 ・・・ Kidney Failure

☐ 腎臓病が懸念されます。直ちに入院していただきたいと思います。

I'm concerned that we're dealing with kidney issues. I'd like to admit you right away.

▶ admit ~（人）：（人）を入院させる

処置・処方

☐ 尿量キットをお渡しします。詳細な指示書が入っているのでそれに従ってください。

I want to give you a urine output kit. There are very specific instructions you'll need to follow.

☐ 1日目、朝起きたら、トイレで排尿してください。その後は、このキットに入っている専用容器を使い、24時間の尿を集めてください。

On day 1, you urinate into the toilet when you get up in the morning. Afterwards, use the special container in this kit and collect your urine for the next 24 hours.

☐ 利尿剤とマンニトールを処方しましょう。

I'm going to put you on diuretics and mannitol.

▶ diuretic：利尿剤　　mannitol：マンニトール　＊脳圧降下剤、乏尿性腎不全の治療薬。

☐ 静脈注射を手配します。

I'm going to order some IV fluids.

▶ IV fluids (intravenous fluids)：静脈注射

☐ 腎生検の予約を入れました。

We've scheduled a kidney biopsy.

▶ kidney biopsy：腎生検

☐ より大きめのサンプルが必要なので、あなたの腎臓の針生検はできません。この生検は外科的に行うことになります。

We need a larger sample, so we can't do a needle biopsy of your kidney. We'll have to do this biopsy surgically.

▶ needle biopsy：針生検

☐ 血液透析と呼ばれる治療を手配します。

I'm going to arrange a medical treatment for you called hemodialysis.

▶ hemodialysis：血液透析

Chapter 4 呼吸器内科

1 慢性閉塞性肺疾患 ●●● COPD

呼吸器内科の Dr. Degawa の診察室にひどい咳を訴える患者が受診しています。彼はちょっとした仕事でも息切れが起きるようです。

Pt. I've been wheezing and coughing a lot. Sometimes I get out of breath just walking up a flight of stairs.

Dr. You said "sometimes." Could you be more specific? How often would you say you have trouble catching your breath?

Pt. I don't know … at least half a dozen times a day, sometimes more. If I'm just sitting around, I'm fine; but even when I'm doing light chores, like washing dishes, I may find myself panting.

Dr. Hmm … how about fatigue?

Pt. Yeah, come to think of it, I'm tired all the time. I used to have a lot more energy.

Dr. Any issue with mucus?

Pt. It seems like I have so much more mucus and phlegm than before.

Dr. You wrote that you're not a smoker. Have you been around smoke or air pollution?

Pt. Some of my family members smoke, so I've had exposure to secondhand smoke.

Dr. I believe you have a condition known as COPD. It's actually a coverall term for a variety of lung diseases, some of which could be serious.

語句・表現

COPD (chronic obstructive pulmonary [pulmonic] disease)：慢性閉塞性肺疾患（医学分野では略語 COPD が一般的に使われている）
wheeze：苦しそうに息をする、ゼーゼー息を切らす
cough：咳をする
get out of breath：息切れがする
flight of stairs：(a ～) 一続きの階段、階と階

1 慢性閉塞性肺疾患 ●●● COPD

訳

P：ゼーゼーと息が切れて咳がひどいのです。ときどき階段を1階分歩いて登っただけで息切れがします。

D：「ときどき」とおっしゃいましたが、もう少し具体的に話していただけますか。どのくらいの頻度で呼吸が苦しくなりますか。

P：よくわかりませんが、少なくとも1日に6回か、それ以上です。ただ座っているだけならよいのですが、皿を洗うといった簡単な雑用をしている時でさえ、息が切れることがあります。

D：うーん。疲れはどうですか。

P：はい、考えてみたら常に疲れています。以前はもっとずっと元気がありました。

D：鼻水はどうですか。

P：前よりも鼻水も痰もとても多いように思います。

D：タバコは吸わないと書いていらっしゃいますね。周囲にタバコを吸う方がいらしたり空気の悪い所にいらっしゃいましたか。

P：家族の何人かはタバコを吸うので、副流煙にさらされてきました。

D：あなたはCOPDとして知られる病状だと思います。実際にはさまざまな重い肺疾患の総称で、その中には重症なものもあります。

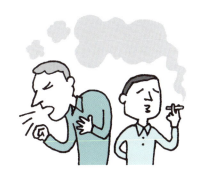

の間の階段
catch one's breath：呼吸が正常に戻る、一息つく
chores：雑用
pant：荒い息をする、息を切らす
mucus：粘液、鼻水
phlegm：痰
secondhand smoke：副流煙

呼吸器内科　使える表現

咳についてたずねる

- **Dr.** 咳の程度はどうですか。
  How bad is the coughing?
  - **Pt.** 本当にひどいのです。咳が始まったら、一息つくのにすら10分程度かかります。
  It's just insane. Once I start coughing, it can take me up to ten minutes to even take a break from the coughing.
    - ▶ insane：常軌を逸した、正気とは思えない

- どのような音の咳ですか。
  What does your cough sound like?

- 咳はどれくらい続いていますか。
  How long have you had the cough?

- 咳をすると痰は出ますか。
  Do you cough up phlegm?

- 薬で咳が静まらないなら、しばらく酸素吸入をする必要があるかもしれません。
  If the medication doesn't calm that down, we may need to put you on oxygen for a while.

呼吸困難についてたずねる

- 呼吸をするのに何か問題がありますか。
  Are you experiencing any difficulty breathing?

- どのくらいの頻度で、呼吸が苦しくなりますか。
  How often would you say you have trouble catching your breath?

- 息切れしますか。
  Do you have shortness of breath?

- 息をするのが難しいですか。
  Do you have difficulty breathing?

1 慢性閉塞性肺疾患 … COPD

☐ 周囲にタバコを吸う方がいらしたり空気の悪い所にいらっしゃいましたか。
❀ Have you been around smoke or air pollution?

診断

☐ あなたはCOPDとして知られる病状だと思います。実際にはさまざまな肺疾患の総称で、その中には重症なものもあります。
❀ I believe you have a condition known as COPD. It's actually a coverall term for a variety of lung diseases, some of which could be serious.

☐ **Pt.** COPDは何の略ですか。
What does COPD stand for?

Dr. Chronic（慢性の）Obstructive（閉塞性の）Pulmonary Disease（肺疾患）です。あなたがそれを、単なるしつこい咳だと思ったとしても、実は肺の病にかかっているのです。

Chronic Obstructive Pulmonary Disease. Even though you thought it was just a lingering cough, you actually have a lung disease.
▶ lingering：なかなか消えない

☐ 咳の様子から見て、慢性気管支炎だろうと思います。
Based on your cough, I'd say this is chronic bronchitis.
▶ bronchitis：気管支炎

☐ あなたは肺気腫です。以前タバコを吸っていらしたのですよね。
You have emphysema. I understand that you used to be a smoker.
▶ emphysema：肺気腫

☐ 喫煙経験者が何年後かに肺気腫を発症するのは珍しくありません。
It isn't unusual for emphysema to show up years later in former smokers.
▶ former smoker：喫煙経験者

☐ あなたは肺気腫にはかかっていないと思います。むしろ数年来の気管支炎が突然、非常に厄介な再発を起こしているのだろうと思います。
I don't think you have emphysema. I'd say you're having a very bad flare-up of the bronchitis you've had for years.
▶ flare-up：突然の再発

医師・臨床医（Clinician）による検査の説明・指示

最大呼気速度（PEFR）

☐ 治療の効果が出ているか、最大呼気速度（PEFR）を測定してみて、あなたのCOPDが改善しているかを見てみましょう。

Let's see if the treatment is effective and your COPD is improving by measuring your peak expiratory flow rate (PEFR).

▶ peak expiratory flow rate (PEFR)：最大呼気速度　ピークフローメーター

トレッドミル運動負荷検査（Treadmill Exercise Test）

運動をしながら行う心電図検査。安静時にはわからない心電図の変化や不整脈・血圧の変化を見て、運動中の心臓の状態を検査します。

☐ トレッドミル（ルームランナー）のスイッチを入れます。

We're turning on the treadmill.

☐ ゆっくりと始めます。ただ歩いてください。だんだんにスピードを上げます。準備はいいですか。

It will start slowly. Just walk with it and we'll gradually increase the speed. Ready?

☐ 結構です。では、2、3分間このチューブで呼吸をしてください。

Good. Now, I want you to breathe into this tube for a couple of minutes.

☐ 次に、血圧を測定したいと思いますが、この検査のため横になってください。

Next, I want to measure your blood pressure, but I'd like you to lie down for this test.

肺機能検査（Pulmonary Function Tests）

☐ いくつか肺機能検査をしたいと思います。最初に、肺活量測定を用いてあなたの肺の容量を分析します。

I'd like to perform some pulmonary function tests. First, we'll analyze your lung capacity using spirometry.

▶ pulmonary function test：肺機能検査
　spirometry：肺活量測定

☐ 機器の使い方を説明します。

Let me show you how to use the device.

☐ 肺活量検査はさまざまな呼吸法を必要とします。

Spirometry tests require various breathing maneuvers.
- ▶ breathing maneuver：呼吸法

☐ まず肺活量(VC)を測定します。これは息をいっぱい吸い込んだあと、肺からどれだけの空気を強制的に吐き出せるかを測ります。

First, we're going to look at your "vital capacity" (VC), how much air you can forcibly exhale from your lungs after a full inhalation.
- ▶ vital capacity (VC)：肺活量
  exhale：息を吐く　　inhalation：吸入

☐ 次は、努力性肺活量(FVC)を測ります。これは、可能な限りこれ以上はできないほどに深く息を吸った後に吐き出す空気量のことです。

Next, we'll look at your "forced vital capacity" (FVC). This is the amount of air that you can exhale after taking the deepest breath you possibly can.
- ▶ forced vital capacity (FVC)：努力性肺活量
  ＊閉塞性疾患の場合には、正常な人とは反対で、肺活量(VC)の方が、努力性肺活量(FVC)よりも大きくなる。

☐ 次に、努力呼出時の最初の1秒間の呼気を調べます。これは努力性呼気1秒量(FEV1)と呼ばれます。

We'll then examine the amount of air that you can forcibly exhale in the first second of forced exhalation, which is called "forced expiratory volume in one second" (FEV1).
- ▶ exhalation：（息などを）吐き出すこと、呼気
  forced expiratory volume in one second：努力性呼気1秒量(FEV1)
  ＊特に閉塞性肺疾患患者の診断とモニタリングに有用。

☐ その後で、努力性肺活量(FVC)に対する努力性呼気1秒量(FEV1)の値を確認したいと思います。

We'll then want to look at your FEV1 to FVC ratio (FEV1/FVC).

☐ 努力呼気流量(FEF)とは、肺からどれだけの空気を吐き出すことができるのかを測定するものです。これは太い気道に閉塞があるかを示すものです。

The "forced expiratory flow" (FEF) measures how much air can be exhaled from the lungs. This is an indicator of large airway obstruction.
- ▶ forced expiratory flow (FEF)：努力呼気流量
  airway obstruction：気道閉塞、気道[気管]障害

Chapter 4 - 呼吸器内科

2　閉塞性睡眠時無呼吸 ●●● OSA

診察室には睡眠障害の患者もよく訪れます。Dr. Degawa は症状を詳しく把握するための検査装置について説明しています。

Dr. It says you have "trouble sleeping." Could you explain this to me in a little more detail?

Pt. I seem to wake up a lot in the night. I spend a lot of time in bed, but I'm always tired.

Dr. I see.

Pt. My wife says that I stop breathing sometimes, too. Actually, she says that I stop breathing long enough that it kind of scares her.

Dr. Have you ever been tested for obstructive sleep apnea?

Pt. No. I actually wondered if that might be what's going on.

Dr. I have a simple home testing unit that you can borrow. Let me ask the nurse to bring it in and I'll explain.

Pt. Is it complicated?

Dr. Not really. There are pictures in this quick guide. We have a long weekend coming up, so go ahead and try it two or three nights, so we can average the data. Why don't you bring it back on Tuesday?

Pt. All right. Will you be able to tell me if I've got sleep apnea then?

Dr. After I look at the data, I'll know if you have a problem. If you have significant disrupted breathing, I'll order a sleep study at a hospital specializing in this for a more precise analysis. These days, OSA is highly treatable, so there's no need for alarm.

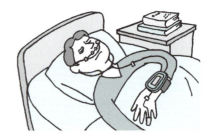

2 閉塞性睡眠時無呼吸 ●●● OSA

訳

D：睡眠障害とのことですね。もう少し詳しく説明していただけますか。

P：夜、何度も起きるようです。かなりの時間を床についていますが、いつも疲れています。

D：なるほど。

P：妻も、私がときどき呼吸を止めていると言います。実は、私が長く息を止めているので、何だか怖くなると言います。

D：閉塞性睡眠時無呼吸の検査をしたことがありますか。

P：いいえ。実は、その症状なのだろうかと思っていました。

D：簡単な自宅での検査装置をお貸しできます。看護師に持ってきてもらって、説明しましょう。

P：複雑ですか。

D：それほどではありません。この簡易ガイドに図があります。長い週末休暇がありますから、2晩か3晩、やってみてください。そうすればデータを平均化できます。火曜日に返却にいらしてはいかがですか。

P：わかりました。そのとき私が睡眠時無呼吸の症状なのかを教えていただくことができますか。

D：データを拝見したら、問題があるかどうかわかるでしょう。呼吸がひどく中断するようなら、より正確な分析を行うために、この症状専門の病院で睡眠検査を手配しましょう。近頃OSAは十分に治療が可能なので、心配することはありません。

語句・表現

obstructive sleep apnea (OSA)：閉塞性睡眠時無呼吸

sleep study：睡眠検査
highly treatable：十分治療可能である

呼吸器内科　使える表現

症状をたずねる

☐ 睡眠障害とのことですね。これについてもう少し詳しく説明していただけますか。

❋ It says you have "trouble sleeping." Could you explain this to me in a little more detail?

☐ 睡眠時に呼吸が止まると言われたことがありますか。

Have you ever been told that you stop breathing while you're asleep?

☐ いびきをかくと言われたことがありますか。

Have you ever been told that you snore?

☐ 仕事中に居眠りが多いですか。

Do you often nod off at work?

検査

☐ 閉塞性睡眠時無呼吸の検査をしたことがありますか。

❋ Have you ever been tested for obstructive sleep apnea?

☐ 長い週末休暇がありますから、2晩か3晩やってみてください。そうすればデータを平均化できます。

❋ We have a long weekend coming up, so go ahead and try it two or three nights, so we can average the data.

CPAP装置

☐ **Dr.** CPAPを使ってみていかがですか。

How are you doing with the CPAP?

Pt. すばらしいです。現在は、一晩中眠っています。

It's great. I'm sleeping through the night, now.

2 閉塞性睡眠時無呼吸 ●●● OSA

☐ **Pt.** CPAP装置を使ってみましたがマスクをつけると閉所恐怖を感じます。

I tried the CPAP machine, but wearing that mask made me feel claustrophobic.

Dr. それを使うのに問題があるわけですね。一部の人にとっての問題は、マスクのサイズです。

I see you're having trouble using it. One issue for some people is the mask size.

▶ claustrophobic：閉所恐怖症の（人）

☐ 明日いらしていただけますか、そうしたらその装置を見てみましょう。

I'd like you to come in tomorrow and let me take a look at it.

☐ **Dr.** 気になっても、その装置を一晩中つけていましたか。

Did you keep it on all night, even though it was bothering you?

Pt. いいえ、真夜中に起きて、また眠ることができなかったので、1、2回で断念しました。

No, I gave up on it one or two times because I woke up in the middle of the night and couldn't get back to sleep.

☐ 眠る前にしばらくマスクをつけておくことをお勧めします。テレビを見たり、何か他のことをしている間にマスクをちょっとつけて、リラックスするよう心がけてください。

One tip is to wear it for a while before you go to sleep. Just put it on while you're watching TV or doing some other activity and try to relax.

Continuous positive airway pressure (CPAP) 持続的気道陽圧法

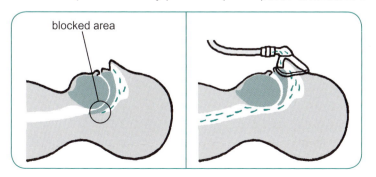

Chapter 5 循環器内科

1 心臓疾患 (1) ●●● Heart Disease

循環器内科のDr. Endoは胸の痛み、立ちくらみ、呼吸困難を訴える患者を診察しています。

CD 2 -08

Dr. Last week, you reported occasional chest pains, lightheadedness and difficulty breathing. Any changes in the symptoms?

Pt. Not really. I'm still having shortness of breath, especially when I lie down in bed.

Dr. I was just going over the results of your echocardiogram. As I suspected, you have MVP.

Pt. MVP?

Dr. It stands for mitral valve prolapse. It's also sometimes called click-murmur syndrome; I think I hear a slight clicking noise when I listen to your heart.

Pt. What causes it to click?

Dr. Basically, the mitral valve in your heart doesn't close tightly. The flaps of the valve are a bit floppy and that causes the symptoms you've been experiencing and the clicking.

Pt. It all sounds very scary.

Dr. Actually, MVP is very common. Many people that have it don't even realize they've got the disease. In your case, since you've been experiencing occasional chest pains, I'd like to prescribe a beta blocker. Let's make you an appointment for a month from now and we can see how it's going.

語句・表現

lightheadedness：頭のふらつき、立ちくらみ
difficulty breathing：呼吸困難
shortness of breath：息切れ
echocardiogram：心エコー図

MVP（mitral valve prolapse）：僧帽弁逸脱
＊僧帽弁逸脱症候群 (mitral valve prolapse syndrome, MVP)：左室収縮期に僧帽弁が左心房内に逸脱 (prolapse) する病態。

1 心臓疾患 (1) ●●● Heart Disease

訳

D：先週あなたは、時折胸の痛み、頭のふらつき、それから呼吸困難を感じるとおっしゃっていましたね。症状に何か変わりはありますか。

P：いいえ、大して変わりません。相変わらず、特に寝室で横になるときに息切れがします。

D：ちょうどあなたの心エコー図の結果を調べたところでした。やはりMVPがあります。

P：MVPとは何ですか。

D：mitral valve prolapse（僧帽弁逸脱）の略です。click-murmur syndrome（クリック音症候群）と呼ばれることもあります。あなたの心臓音を聞くと、わずかなカチっという音が聞こえるでしょう。

P：何がカチっという音を引き起こすのでしょうか。

D：基本的には、心臓の僧帽弁がしっかりと閉じていないために起こります。弁の蓋が少し弱くなっており、それがあなたの症状や、クリック音を引き起こすのです。

P：すべてがとても恐ろしく思えます。

D：実はMVPは非常に一般的な病気です。この病状を持つ多くの人が、そうした病気を持っていることにすら気付いていません。あなたの場合は、時折胸の痛みを経験しているので、ベータ・ブロッカー（心臓薬）を処方したいと思います。今日から1ヶ月後の予約を取って、経過を見ましょう。

---

click-murmur syndrome：クリック音症候群（僧帽弁逸脱と同義）
clicking noise：カチッという音
mitral valve：僧帽弁
flap：蓋（ふた）

floppy：やわらかい、弱い
beta blocker：β（ベータ）ブロッカー、遮断薬（心臓薬、交感神経薬）

循環器内科　使える表現

症状をたずねる

☐ 不整脈があると診断されたことがありますか。
Have you ever been diagnosed with an irregular heartbeat?

☐ 時折胸の痛みや頭のふらつき、呼吸困難を感じるとおっしゃっていましたね。症状に何か変化はありますか。
❋ You reported occasional chest pains, lightheadedness and difficulty breathing. Any changes in the symptoms?

☐ **Dr.** ここに、頻繁に胸焼けがする、とありますが。
It says here that you have frequent heartburn.
Pt. はい、その症状は何年にもなります。昔ほど頻繁ではありませんが、先日のものはひどかったです。
Yes, I've had it for years. It isn't as frequent as it used to be, but it was bad the other day.
▶ have heartburn：胸焼けがする

☐ **Dr.** 頻繁に胸焼けが起こるのですね。それは食事をとった直後に起こりますか。
You've been suffering from frequent heartburn? Does it occur soon after you've had a meal?
Pt. はい、いつも食事の後だと思います。
Yes, I'd say it's always after a meal.

☐ **Dr.** 胸焼けは起き上がったらよくなりましたか。
Did your heartburn get better once you sat up?

診察・診断

☐ あなたの心臓音を聞くと、わずかなカチっという音が聞こえるでしょう。
❋ I think I hear a slight clicking noise when I listen to your heart.

☐ では、心電図をとってみましょう。
I'd like to get an electrocardiogram now.

☐ これは心膜炎あるいは狭心症の可能性があります。胸のX線と心電図の手配から始めたいと思います。
This could be pericarditis or angina. I'd like to start by ordering

a chest X-ray and an EKG.
> pericarditis：心膜炎　　angina：狭心症
> EKG = elektrokardiogramm：（ドイツ語）心電図
> ＊ECG=electrocardiogram：（英語）心電図

☐ 心音は正常です。あなたはとても若いので、標準的な胸焼け、あるいは初期の胃酸の逆流だろうと思います。

Your heart sounds normal. You're quite young, so I suspect this is classic heartburn, or possibly the beginning of acid reflux.
> acid reflux：（胃）酸の逆流

負荷検査

☐ 症状から（心臓の）負荷検査を行うことにしました。検査装置を付けていただき、心臓が一定量の運動をどの程度こなすかを測定します。

Based on your symptoms, I've decided to do a stress test. We need to hook you up and monitor how well your heart handles certain activity.
> stress test：負荷検査　　hook ～ up：（機器などに）～を接続する

☐ リラックスしてください。この検査で、血液を心臓に運ぶ動脈の血液の供給が実際に減少しているかどうかがわかります。

Try to relax. This test shows us exactly whether or not the blood supply is reduced in the arteries that supply blood to the heart.

☐ この検査は、今後どのくらいの運動をこなすことができるかということも示してくれます。

It will also give us an idea how much exercise you will be able to handle in the future.

☐ この検査は「心血管造影検査」と呼ばれるもので、あなたの心臓の大きさと形を調べることができます。

This one is called a "nuclear stress test" and will let us look at the size and shape of your heart.
> nuclear stress test：心血管造影検査

☐ 「駆出率」と呼ばれる心臓のポンプ機能も測ることもできます。

We'll also be able to measure the pumping function, which is called the "ejection fraction."
> ejection fraction：駆出率

Chapter 5 - 循環器内科

2　心臓疾患 (2) ●●● Heart Disease

ER から心拍数 130 の患者が運ばれました。Dr. Endo は脳卒中の恐れがあると判断します。

Dr. The ER says you came in with lightheadedness and a <u>heart rate</u> of 130. How are you feeling now? Any chest pain or <u>shortness of breath</u>?

Pt. No.

P.W. (Patient's wife): He said he felt like he was going to <u>faint</u>.

Dr. Hmm … <u>presyncope</u> … I believe we're looking at an <u>atrial flutter</u> here. When the heart rate is elevated and unstable, there's a <u>risk of stroke</u>. I'd like to do a cardioversion. We'll use this to shock your heart back into normal <u>sinus rhythm</u>.

Pt. Oh, like you see on TV?

Dr. I'm actually going to let the machine do the work. We won't be standing over you with paddles. The nurse will be right back to run an <u>intravenous line</u>. I'm going to give you a mild <u>anesthetic</u>, but <u>chances are</u> you will still feel the shock. In other words, it's still going to hurt a little.

(pause)

Dr. Okay, Mrs. Miller, I need you to step aside and <u>stay clear of</u> the wires.

Pt. Yes, honey, Clear! I've always wanted to say that …

Dr. If you're joking you must be feeling a little better. I'm glad you're in a good mood. Because we're treating this as an emergency, we're keeping you somewhat alert for this. Charging to 200…

語句・表現

heart rate：心拍数
shortness of breath：息切れ
faint：気絶する、失神する
presyncope：失神寸前の状態

atrial flutter：心房粗動（不整脈の一種）
risk of stroke：脳卒中のリスク
cardioversion：電気的除細動
sinus rhythm：サイナスリズム（洞調律）

2 心臓疾患 (2) ●●● Heart Disease

訳

D：ER（緊急治療室）によると、あなたは、立ちくらみと心拍数130で運ばれたとのことですが。今気分はいかがですか。胸の痛み、あるいは息切れはありますか。

P：いいえ。

P（患者の妻）：夫は意識を失うように感じると言っていました。

D：うーん。失神寸前の状態ですね…。心房粗動だと思います。心拍数が上がり不安定だと、脳卒中のリスクがあります。電気的除細動を行いたいと思います。この装置を使って、心臓にショックを与えて正常なサイナスリズムに戻します。

P：ああ、テレビ番組で見るような処置ですか。

D：実は、これから装置を動かすところです。私たちはパドルを持ってあなたのそばに立つことはしません。看護師がすぐに戻ってきて、静脈ラインを確保します。軽い麻酔を打ちますが、それでもショックを感じるでしょう。つまり、少し痛みを感じるということです。

（中断）

D：いいですか、ミラーさん、脇へ寄ってワイヤーに近づかないでください。

P：いいかい、君。離れて！　僕はいつもそう言ってみたかったんだ。

D：あなたが冗談をおっしゃっているならば、少し気分がよくなっているのでしょう。気分がよくてよかったです。私たちは、緊急措置として対処しているため、（麻酔をかけたと言っても）あなたには幾らか意識をしっかり持った状態でいていただくことになるからです。除細動装置を200に合わせます。

＊洞結節で発生した電気的興奮が正しく心臓全体に伝わり、心臓が正常なリズムを示している状態。

intravenous line：静脈ライン

anesthetic：麻酔薬

chances are (that) ~：おそらく~だろう、ひょっとしたら~

stay clear of ~：~に近づかない

Chapter 5 循環器内科

循環器内科　使える表現

症状をたずねる

☐ 胸の痛み、あるいは息切れはありますか。
Do you have any chest pain or shortness of breath?

☐ 意識を失うように感じたことはありますか。
Have you felt like you were going to faint?

☐ 立ちくらみをしたことがありますか。
Have you experienced any lightheadedness?

☐ 心拍数が上がり不安定だと、脳卒中のリスクがあります。
❉ When the heart rate is elevated and unstable, there's a risk of stroke.

処置・処方

● 電気的除細動

☐ 電気的除細動を行いたいと思います。この装置を使って、心臓にショックを与えて正常なサイナスリズムに戻します。

❉ I'd like to do a cardioversion. We'll use this to shock your heart back into normal sinus rhythm.

☐ 軽い麻酔を打ちますが、それでもあなたはショックを感じるかもしれません。

❉ I'm going to give you a mild anesthetic, but chances are you will still feel the shock.

☐ プリントアウトをお見せしましょう。あなたの心臓の鼓動が非常に速かったときの、スパイクの波形をこれで確認できます。

Let me show you the printout. Here you can see what the spikes were like when your heart was beating so fast.

▶ spike：スパイク（パルス波形の一部分で発生する瞬時過渡現象）

☐ あなたの心臓が正常に鼓動し始めたのがわかるでしょう。
You'll notice where your heart started beating normally.

2 心臓疾患 (2) ●●● Heart Disease

☐ このモニターを見てください。今あなたの心臓は正常なサイナスリズムですよ。

Look at the monitor. Your heart is in normal sinus rhythm now.

●埋め込み式ループレコーダー

☐ 私はあなたが原因不明の失神発作、つまり気絶を何度か発症していらっしゃることが気にかかっています。

I'm concerned that you've had several episodes of unexplained syncope, in other words, fainting.

▶ unexplained syncope：原因不明の失神

☐ 非常に簡単な外科的治療を行いたいと思います。埋め込み式ループレコーダーをあなたの胸につけて、あなたの心臓をモニターします。

I'd like to do a very simple surgical procedure. We put an implantable loop recorder in your chest to monitor your heart.

▶ implantable loop recorder (ILR)：埋め込み式ループレコーダー

☐ 埋め込み式ループレコーダー (ILR) を装着したので、1ヶ月後に再診してください。そうすれば、私はさまざまな測定値を得て、どの状態にあるかが確認できます。

Now that you have the ILR, I want you to come back in a month. Then I can get various readings and see where we're at.

▶ readings：測定値、数値

☐ さらに症状が出た場合は、必ず、直ちに私たちに連絡してください。

You should be in touch with us right away if you have any further episodes.

●ペースメーカー

☐ あなたには例えば、倒れて頭を打つ危険性が常にあるのです。ペースメーカーはあなたの心臓を正常に維持するでしょう。

You're in constant danger of falling and hitting your head, for example. The pacemaker will keep your heart on track.

☐ あなたの心臓は、除脈性と頻脈性の不整脈を交互に発症しています。最善の治療方法は、ペースメーカーを取り付けることだと思います。

Your heart alternates between slow arrhythmias and fast arrhythmias. We think the best solution is to put in a pacemaker.

▶ arrhythmias：不整脈　　slow arrhythmia：徐脈性不整脈
fast arrhythmia：頻脈性不整脈

Chapter 5 循環器内科

3 高血圧症 ●●● High Blood Pressure

循環器内科の Dr. Endo の診察室を定期的に受診している患者は、病院に来ると血圧が高くなるようです。

Dr. Hi, how are you today?

Pt. Fine, thanks.

Dr. I'd like to check your blood pressure. It's been on the high side the last few times. … hmm, it's 143 over 80.

Pt. It's not usually that high. This seems to happen when I'm in the doctor's office.

Dr. Ah, it sounds like you have white coat syndrome.

Pt. Is that really a thing?

Dr. It's quite common, actually. It's also called "white coat hypertension," when discussed among doctors. I want to make sure that that's all this is. So, I want to recommend that you get a home monitoring kit and take your blood pressure a few times a day.

Pt. Actually, I think my mother-in-law has one I can borrow.

Dr. All right. Why don't you create a little diary and write down the numbers every day for the next ten days and plan to see me again after that.

Pt. Could you remind me what the ideal numbers are?

Dr. If you're under 120 systolic, the top number, and under 80, diastolic, the bottom number, that's fantastic. If you're somewhat higher than that, it's not a big problem, but if you're considerably higher, like what we saw with your systolic number today, we might consider medication.

語句・表現

on the high[low] side：高め[低め]で
white coat syndrome, white coat hypertension：白衣高血圧（症）
systolic：（心臓の）収縮の
diastolic：心臓拡張の

3 高血圧症 ●●● High Blood Pressure

訳

D：こんにちは、今日はいかがですか。

P：順調です、ありがとうございます。

D：血圧を測りたいと思います。ここ2、3回、高めです。うーん、143と80ですね。

P：いつもはそんなに高くありません。このことは、病院にいると起こる気がします。

D：ああ、あなたは「白衣高血圧（white coat syndrome）」のようですね。

P：本当にそんなことがあるのですか。

D：これは実は極めてよく起こることなのです。医師の間で話すときには「white coat hypertension」とも呼ばれています。この（血圧の高さが）白衣高血圧のものであるかを確かめたいと思います。ですので、家庭用モニターキットを入手して、1日に数回血圧を測ることをお勧めします。

P：実は、義理の母が持っているものを借りられると思います。

D：わかりました。ちょっとした日記帳を作り、これから10日間、毎日数値を書き留めてみてください。その後、また受診を予定してください。

P：理想的な血圧の数値はどれくらいでしたでしょうか。

D：心収縮期の血圧、最大血圧が120以下で、心拡張期の血圧、最小血圧が80以下であれば理想的です。それよりもいくらか高めならばたいした問題ではありませんが、今日の心収縮期の数値のようにかなり高ければ、投薬を検討するかもしれません。

雑学
White Coat Hypertension（白衣高血圧）と Masked Hypertension（仮面高血圧）

　会話では「白衣高血圧」を扱いましたが、白衣高血圧とは正反対の状態で、「仮面高血圧」という症状があります。これは、診察室や病院では正常血圧とされるために本当の高血圧がマスクされるという意味で、「仮面をかぶった（masked）」が使われています。

　最近では病院で測るよりも家庭血圧の方が高い「仮面高血圧」が「白衣高血圧」よりも脳梗塞や心筋梗塞を発症させるリスクが高いことがわかってきました。どちらのタイプも、発見には家庭での血圧測定が不可欠です。

循環器内科　使える表現

血圧測定

☐ 血圧を測りたいと思います。ここ2、3回、高めです。143と80ですね。

✢ I'd like to check your blood pressure. It's been on the high side the last few times. It's 143 over 80.

☐ 1、2分静かに座って、深く息を吸ってください。あなたが落ち着いていらっしゃれば、より正確な数値が測れます。

Please sit quietly for a minute or two, taking deep breaths. I'll get a more accurate reading if you're calm.
▶ reading：（計測器などの）測定値、示度数、表示数値

☐ そこに座って、その機械を使っていただけますか。

Could you sit over there and use the machine?

☐ **Pt.** 今までそれを使ったことがありません。どうしたらいいですか。

I've never used one before, what do I do?

N 手のひらを上に向けてただ腕を通していただくだけです。その後、スタートボタンを押してください。

Just put your arm through with your palm facing up. Then, push the start button.

☐ 家庭用モニターキットを入手して、1日に数回血圧を測ることをお勧めします。

✢ I want to recommend that you get a home monitoring kit and take your blood pressure a few times a day.

診断・処方

☐ 以前血圧が高いと言われたことがありますか。

Were you ever told that your blood pressure was high before?

☐ 心収縮期の血圧、最大血圧が120以下で、心拡張期の血圧、最小血圧が80以下であれば理想的です。

✢ If you are under 120 systolic, the top number, and under 80, diastolic, the bottom number, that's fantastic.

☐ あなたの血圧は正常よりやや高めですね。

Your blood pressure is a little above normal.

3 高血圧症 ● ● ● High Blood Pressure

☐ ご自身のモニタリングとこれまでの診察の間に観察してきた数値からすると、あなたはステージ1の高血圧症だと思います。

Based on your self-monitoring and the numbers we have seen during your appointments, I believe you have stage 1 hypertension.

▸ hypertension=high blood pressure：高血圧症

☐ **Pt.** 私はどう対応すべきでしょうか。

What should I do about it?

Dr. ナトリウムの摂取を減らしていただきたいと思います。少量の薬を処方しましょう。

I'd like you to cut down on your sodium intake. I'm going to prescribe a small dose of medication.

☐ あなたの測定値は160台です。これはステージ2の高血圧症だということですので、しばらく投薬をしたいと思います。

Your readings have been in the 160s. This means you have stage 2 hypertension, so I'd like to put you on medication for a while.

☐ 観察を続けて、あなたが適度な運動と食事をすれば、数ヶ月で投薬を止めることができるかもしれません。

We can keep monitoring it and if you exercise and eat properly, we may be able to wean you off of it in a few months.

▸ wean off：〜をやめさせる

高血圧症がもたらすダメージ (Damage from high blood pressure may include)

stroke：脳卒中	blindness：失明	heart attack：心臓発作
heart failure：心不全	kidney failure：腎不全	

血圧測定値分類 (The American Heart Association 使用)

Blood Pressure Category 血圧分類	Systolic 心収縮期（最大） mm Hg (upper #)		Diastolic 心拡張期（最小） mm Hg (lower #)
Normal　平常	Less than 120	and	Less than 80
Prehypertension　前高血圧症	120 - 139	or	80 - 89
Hypertension - Stage 1　軽症	140 - 159	or	90 - 99
Hypertension - Stage 2　中等症	160 or higher	or	100 or higher
Hypertensive Crisis（高血圧クライシス／緊急の措置を要する）	Higher than 180	or	Higher than 110

Chapter 5 - 循環器内科

4 動脈硬化 ●●● Arteriosclerosis

循環器内科の Dr. Endo は手足にしびれを感じて受診した患者を診察します。自分の症状をあまり深刻には捉えていなかったようです。

Dr. It says here you've been experiencing weakness and numbness in your extremities. I'd like to listen to your heart. I'm hearing something that may be bruits.

Pt. Bruits?

Dr. I think I hear a whooshing noise over your arteries. This is the kind of sound that occurs when the blood is having to work to pass over some sort of obstruction. I think we may be dealing with arteriosclerosis here.

Pt. So my heart is bad?

Dr. It's likely that you have a build-up of plaque in your arteries.

Pt. Oh …

Dr. Let's do some imaging. I'd like to get an electrocardiogram and I also want to use ultrasound to see what kind of blockages might be occurring along your arms and legs. I'd like to have you fast for nine to twelve hours and come in for a blood test. We can check your blood sugar and cholesterol to see what's going on.

Pt. I can't believe I have hardening of the arteries. I'm not that old.

Dr. Well, there are some lifestyle changes you can make right off the bat. I'd like you to do some mild exercise every day and avoid foods high in fat and salt. Let's see what the results of these tests are.

語句・表現

arteriosclerosis：動脈硬化
weakness：脱力感
extremities：手足（四肢）
bruit：雑音
whooshing noise：シュッ（ヒュー）という雑音

obstruction：閉塞、障害
electrocardiogram：心電図
ultrasound：超音波
blockage：閉塞
fast：食を控える
hardening：硬化

4 動脈硬化 ●●● Arteriosclerosis

訳

D: これを読むと、あなたは手足に脱力感やしびれを経験しているようですね。心臓の音を聞かせてください。何か雑音のようなものが聞こえます。

P: 雑音ですか。

D: 動脈にシュッ（ヒュー）という雑音が聞こえるように思います。これは血液が、何らかの障害を通り過ぎようとして作用するときに起こる類の音です。ここの動脈硬化に対処することになるかと思います。

P: では、私の心臓が悪いと。

D: あなたの動脈内に、血小板の塊が形成されているようです。

P: なんということ…

D: いくつか画像検査をしましょう。心電図をとり、それから超音波も使用して、どんな種類の閉塞があなたの腕や足に起きているのか確認したいと思います。9時間から12時間、食事を控えてから、血液検査に来ていただきたいと思います。血糖値とコレステロールを検査し、状態を確認したいので。

P: 私に動脈硬化があるなんて信じられません。私はそんなに年をとっていませんよ。

D: ええと、あなたが今すぐに行える生活習慣の変更がいくつかあります。毎日、いくらか軽い運動を行い、脂肪や塩分の多い食事を控えていただきたいと思います。検査の結果を確認しましょう。

動脈硬化の考えられる原因	Causes of arteriosclerosis
・高脂肪食、高コレステロール	・High-fat diets and cholesterol
・喫煙	・Smoking
・高血圧	・High blood pressure
・動脈硬化または心臓病の家族歴	・A family history of arteriosclerosis or heart disease
・活動的でない生活習慣	・An inactive lifestyle
・肥満	・Overweight or obesity
・糖尿病	・Diabetes
・アルコール	・Alcohol
・大気汚染	・Air pollution

循環器内科　使える表現

症状をたずねる

☐ 体の末端の部分、つまりあなたの手足に脱力感やしびれを感じますか。

Have you been feeling any weakness or numbness in your extremities ... I mean in your arms and legs?

☐ 歩いていると、太ももやふくらはぎに痛みを感じますか。

Are you experiencing any pain in your thighs or calves when you walk?

☐ 階段を上り下りすると動悸がしますか。

Do you ever experience shortness of breath when you go up and down the stairs?

☐ 重い荷物を持って歩くと息苦しくなりますか。

Do you ever experience shortness of breath when you carry something heavy?

☐ アザができやすいですか。傷ができると治らず化膿したり膿が出たりしますか。

Are you bruising easily? Do you have wounds that don't heal or develop pus or a dishcharge?

診察

☐ 心臓の音を聞かせてください。何か雑音のようなものが聞こえます。

🩺 I'd like to listen to your heart. I'm hearing something that may be bruits.

☐ 動脈にシュッ（ヒュー）という雑音が聞こえます。

🩺 I hear a whooshing noise over your arteries.

☐ あなたの動脈内に、血小板の塊が形成されているようです

🩺 It's likely that you have a build-up of plaque in your arteries.

☐ 検査の結果は、あなたの血糖値とコレステロール値が高いことを示しています。

Your test results show that both your blood sugar and cholesterol are high.

4 動脈硬化 ... Arteriosclerosis

□ しばらく動脈硬化の薬を投与なさっていますね。βブロッカーを服用されているのですね。

You've been taking medication for arteriosclerosis for a while. I see you've been on a beta blocker.

▶ beta blocker：β（ベータ）ブロッカー［遮断薬］（心臓薬、交感神経薬）

保存的な治療（Conservative Treatment）

□ 私たちはあなたの動脈硬化症に取り組んでいきます。まず、あなたのコレステロール値を大幅に下げる薬の服用から始めましょう。

We need to address your arteriosclerosis. Let's start with some medication that should drastically lower your cholesterol.

□ 少し生活習慣を変えることをお勧めします。

I recommend you make some lifestyle changes.

□ 毎日いくらか軽い運動を行い、脂肪や塩分の多い食事を控えてください。

❂ I'd like you to do some mild exercise every day and avoid foods high in fat and salt.

積極的な治療（Aggressive Treatment）

□ 症状はあまり改善されていないようなので、もう少し積極的な治療を行いたいと思います。

It seems that your condition hasn't improved, so I'd like to be a little more aggressive with your treatment.

□ 心臓カテーテル手術を受けていただきたいと思います。

I'd like you to have a cardiac catheterization.

▶ cardiac catheterization：心臓カテーテル法

□ 日本は、世界で最も心臓カテーテル手術の割合が高い国の一つです。あなたにはそうした手術を受けるのが適していると思います。

Japan has one of the highest percentages of cardiac catheterization in the world. I think you'd be a good candidate for that sort of a procedure.

□ **Pt.** 心臓カテーテル手術で何が引き起こされますか。

What does the cardiac catheterization entail?

Dr. あなたにそのことを説明するよう、外科医に頼んでおきます。

I'll ask the surgeon to explain it to you.

▶ entail：～を引き起こす、伴う

心臓カテーテル手術の手順（Cardiac Catheterization Procedure）

カテーテル挿入

☐ 手順は極めて簡単です。麻酔科医があなたの手首に麻酔をかけたら、私は病巣となる動脈の部分に誘導されたガイドワイヤーに従って、前腕にある橈骨（とうこつ）動脈にシースを挿入します。

This procedure is remarkably simple. The anesthesiologist will numb your wrist and I'll insert a sheath into the radial artery in your forearm, followed by a guide wire that will be maneuvered up to the area of the diseased artery.

▶ anesthesiologist：麻酔科医　　numb：（人の）感覚をなくする、まひさせる
　sheath：シース（カテーテルを体内に挿入する際に通り道となる管）
　radial artery：橈骨（とうこつ）動脈（手首にある血管）
　forearm：前腕

☐ ガイドワイヤーは、私がカテーテルを正しい部位へとうまく誘導する手助けとなります。

The guide wire will help me move the catheter smoothly to the right place.

☐ カテーテルが所定の位置に入ったら、ガイドワイヤーを取り除き、カテーテルをさまざまなツールとなる導管として使うことができます。

Once the catheter is in place, I'll remove the guide wire and I'll be able to use the catheter as a conduit for various tools.

▶ conduit：導管

ロータブレーター

☐ あなたの場合は、まずロータブレーターと呼ばれる特別な装置を先端に使います。ロータブレーターは、ダイヤモンドが先端についたドリルで、1分間に約21万回転します。

In your case, first I'll use a special fitting on the end, called a "rotablator," which is a diamond-tipped drill that spins at about 210,000 revolutions per minute.

▶ rotablator：ロータブレーター（動脈硬化組織を削る装置）

☐ 私はこの装置を使って、あなたの動脈を閉塞している石灰化プラークに穴を空けて削り取ります。実際には、血小板を取り除くのにわずか2、3秒しかかかりません。

This will let me drill through and shave off the calcified plaque that is blocking your artery. Actually, it will take just a few seconds to remove the plaque.

▶ calcified plaque：石灰化プラーク

ステントの挿入

- [ ] その後、カテーテルを使って、ステントを挿入します。

    After that, I'll insert a stent, which is a 20mm tube made of stainless steel, through the catheter.

    ▶ stent：ステント（ステンレス鋼でできた20mmのチューブで、血管、気管などの狭窄部を内部から広げる管状の機器）

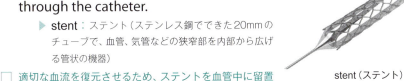

stent（ステント）

- [ ] 適切な血流を復元させるため、ステントを血管中に留置します。

    This is deployed inside your blood vessel to restore the proper flow of blood.

- [ ] これが終わったら、ステントを拡張するために高い圧力への抵抗性を持つバルーンを挿入するという、最後のステップに進みます。

    That is followed by the last step, where I insert a high pressure-resistant balloon to expand the stent.

    ▶ high pressure-resistant：高圧力抵抗性の

- [ ] このようにして、ステントを動脈の壁にしっかり適合させるのです。

    This will make the stent hug the artery wall.

血管のステント治療

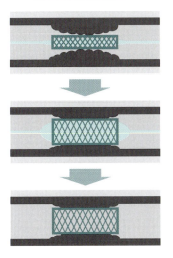

Inserting a balloon
（バルーンを挿入する）

Expandingt the stent
（ステントを拡張させる）

Pulling out the balloon to restore the proper flow of blood
（バルーンを取り出して適切な血流を復元させる）

Chapter 6 - 血液内科

1 リンパ腫 ●●● Lymphoma

血液内科の Dr. Fujita の診察室を受診した患者には、発熱、発汗に加え、脇の下や腹部に痛みがあります。

Dr. You say you've had night sweats, fevers and abdominal pain? Let's do a brief physical. The nurse got your weight today, right?

Pt. Yes, she took my weight. I'm down about three kilos, but I haven't been dieting.

Dr. Do you get full very quickly after eating just a small amount?

Pt. Yeah, come to think of it. It seems like I just begin a meal and I find myself full in a minute or two.

Dr. I'd like to see if your lymph nodes are at all swollen. Let's have you lie down on the table on your back with your arms at your sides.

Pt. Umm … sure. (pause) Ow …

Dr. So it's tender here under your arms, then?

Pt. Yes, but only when you touch it.

Dr. What about if I push on your stomach here?

Pt. That really hurts.

Dr. I do detect some swelling of your lymph nodes. Because of some of the other symptoms, I'd like to schedule an MRI. Depending on the results, we may need to do a biopsy. Right now, I'd like to send you to the second floor for some blood tests.

Pt. So this means it's quite serious?

Dr. We won't know anything for sure until we analyze the tissue. I think I can get you in this week, so we can get some answers back sooner rather than later.

1 リンパ腫 ●●● Lymphoma

訳

D：寝汗、発熱それに腹痛があるとのことですね。簡単な身体検査をしましょう。看護師が今日のあなたの体重を測りましたね。

P：はい、体重を測ってもらいました。約3キロ減っていますが、ダイエットはしていません。

D：ほんの少しの量で食後すぐに満腹になりますか。

P：考えてみれば、そうです。食事を始めて、1、2分で満腹を感じます。

D：リンパ節がまず腫れ上がっているか調べたいと思います。その台の上に、両腕を脇につけてあおむけに寝てください。

P：ええ…わかりました。痛い！

D：なるほど、両腕の下のここが触ると痛いのですね、これはどうですか。

P：はい、でも先生が触ったときだけです。

D：腹部のここを押すとどうですか。

P：とても痛いです。

D：いくつかのリンパ節に腫れが見られます。他のいくつかの症状を確認するため、MRIの予定を入れたいと思います。検査の結果次第で、生検を行う必要があるかもしれません。今すぐ、2階でいくつか血液検査を受けていただきたいと思います。

P：それで、これはかなり深刻な症状でしょうか。

D：組織を分析するまでは、何もはっきりしたことはわかりません。結果を今週中に入手できると思うので、割合早く病状についてのお答えをお知らせできるでしょう。

語句・表現

abdominal pain：腹痛
do a physical：身体検査をする
lymph nodes：リンパ節
with one's arms at one's sides：両腕を脇につけて
tender：圧痛のある、触ると痛い
biopsy：バイオプシー、生体組織検査（生検）

＊生体の組織や臓器の一部を採取して、病気を診断する検査のこと。悪性腫瘍が疑われる患者に行われることが多く、皮膚や胃、腸、肝臓、肺、腎臓などの組織を使って診断される。

sooner rather than later：割合早く、割合すぐに、すぐにでも

血液内科　使える表現

診察

☐ しこりが感じ取れるとのことですね。
You say you can feel a lump?

☐ リンパ節がまず腫れ上がっているか調べたいと思います。
❀ I'd like to see if your lymph nodes are at all swollen.

☐ その台の上に、両腕を脇につけてあおむけに寝てください。
❀ Let's have you lie down on the table on your back with your arms at your sides.

☐ 正確にどこにあるのか見せてください。
Show me exactly where you feel this.

☐ 腹部のここを押すとどうですか。
❀ What about if I push on your stomach here?

☐ いくつかのリンパ節に腫れが見られます。
❀ I do detect some swelling of your lymph nodes.

病歴をたずねる

☐ 自己免疫疾患にかかったことはありますか。
Is there any history of autoimmune disease?
　▶ autoimmune disease：自己免疫疾患（AID）

☐ 肝臓の病気はどうですか。肝炎にかかったことはありますか。
What about liver issues? Have you ever had hepatitis?
　▶ hepatitis：肝臓炎、肝炎

☐ 農薬や殺虫剤がかかる環境にあったことはありますか。
Have you been around pesticides or insecticides?
　▶ pesticide：農薬　　insecticide：殺虫剤

☐ その種の毒素はリンパ腫の主な危険因子と考えられています。
Those types of toxins are suspected to be a major risk factor for lymphoma.

1 リンパ腫 ●●● Lymphoma

診断・処置

☐ がんは1つの可能性ですが、これは何かの感染によるものかもしれません。

Cancer is a possibility, but this can sometimes be from some sort of infection.

☐ 2週間抗生剤を服用していただきたいのです。しこりが消えれば、たぶんがんの検査をすることはないでしょう。

I want you to do a two-week course of antibiotics. If it goes away, then we are probably not looking at a cancer.
  ▶ antibiotics：抗生剤

☐ 残念ながらバイオプシー（生検）の結果はあなたが非ホジキンリンパ腫であることを示しています。

I'm sorry to say that the biopsy indicates that you do have non-Hodgkin's lymphoma.
  ▶ non-Hodgkin('s) lymphoma (NHL)：非ホジキンリンパ腫（ホジキン病以外の悪性リンパ腫の総称）

☐ CBC（完全血球算定）ならびに血液化学検査で腎臓と肝臓機能をチェックし、それからLDH（乳酸脱水素酵素）検査を行います。

We'd like to get a CBC, complete blood count, as well as blood chemistry tests, to check your kidney and liver function, and an LDH test.
  ▶ CBC (complete blood count)：完全血球算定
     LDH (lactate dehydrogenase)：乳酸脱水素酵素

☐ 病状がバイオプシーで採取した1カ所に限られているならば、これはまだ第1ステージだということです。

If we find that the disease is limited to the one area where we took the biopsy, it will mean that this is still in Stage 1.

☐ 症状が広がっておらず、血清のLDHレベルが平常値ならば予後診断は極めて良好です。

The prognosis is very good if the disease has not spread and the serum LDH level is normal.
  ▶ prognosis：予後（診断）　　serum：血清

Chapter 6 血液内科

2 悪性貧血 ●●● Pernicious Anemia

胃の具合が悪いと女性患者がDr. Fujitaの診察を受けています。症状を詳しくたずねてみると、米国で医師から貧血の疑いを示唆されていたようです。 CD2-13

Dr. Today's visit has something to do with stomach trouble?

Pt. Yes, I do have stomach trouble, but I'm concerned that this is something else. I went to see my doctor in Indiana last month. I was having issues with frequent diarrhea. She started talking about doing blood tests for some sort of anemia.

Dr. Ah … I see now. Let's go step by step. Do you have any other symptoms besides diarrhea?

Pt. I don't feel like doing much these days. I was never this lethargic before.

Dr. Well, if you have pernicious anemia, diarrhea and lethargy are possible symptoms. Pale skin is another symptom.

Pt. I don't know what kind of anemia that is. I had a bit of an iron deficiency when I was in my 20s, but I'm in my 50s now. I'm no longer menstruating.

Dr. This type of anemia affects people over 30. It is actually most common in people around 60. This type of anemia is about not being able to absorb vitamin B-12 from your intestines. Let's start out with a CBC and look at all of the ordinary levels in your blood.

語句・表現

lethargic：無気力な、不活発な
iron deficiency：鉄欠乏
menstruating：月経中の
vitamin B-12：ビタミンB12

CBC (complete blood (cell) count)：完全血球算定
＊採取した血液中の赤血球と白血球と血小板の数を調べる検査法。

2 悪性貧血 ●●● Pernicious Anemia

訳

D：今日は胃の具合が悪くていらしたのですね。

P：はい、胃の具合が悪いのですが、何か他の病気があるのではと心配しています。先月インディアナで、かかりつけの医師の診察を受けました。私は始終下痢に悩まされていました。ドクターからは何らかの貧血の可能性を調べるための血液検査を行うことを提案されていたところです。

D：ああ、今わかりました。少しずつ進めましょう。下痢以外に何か他の症状はありますか。

P：最近、あまりやる気が出ません。こうした無気力感は今までまったくありませんでした。

D：ええと、あなたが悪性貧血だとすれば、下痢や無気力感はありうる症状です。顔色が青白いのもその症状です。

P：これがどんな種類の貧血なのかわかりません。私は20代の時に少し鉄欠乏症でしたが、今は50代です。もう月経はありませんし。

D：この種の貧血は30歳過ぎの人々がかかりますが、実は60歳前後の方々に最もよく見られるものです。この種の貧血は、腸からビタミンB12を吸収することができないことによるものです。完全血球算定から始めて、血中のあらゆる項目のレベルを調べましょう。

雑学
網状赤血球（レチクロ）数算定

reticulocyte count (retic count)、reticulocyte percent とも言います。

網状赤血球は幼若な赤血球で、赤血球中に含まれる RNA（リボ核酸）が検査で染色されると網状に見えることから網状赤血球と言います。約1〜2日で脾臓でRNAが取り除かれ、成熟した赤血球となります。短期間で成熟赤血球となるため、網赤血球数の増加・減少を検査することで、骨髄の赤血球産生能力が測れます。

● 網状赤血球（レチクロ）数が異常な場合に疑われる病気

高値…溶血性貧血　　　　hemolytic anemia
　　　鉄欠乏性貧血　　　iron-deficiency anemia
　　　巨赤芽球性貧血　　megaloblastic anemia など
低値…再生不良性貧血　　aplastic anemia
　　　骨髄線維症　　　　myelofibrosis
　　　急性白血病　　　　acute leukemia など

血液内科　使える表現

貧血

☐ 顔色が悪いと言われたことがありますか。

Has anyone told you that you look pale?

☐ 下痢以外に何か他の症状はありますか。

🍀 Do you have any other symptoms besides diarrhea?

☐ 顔色が青白いのはもう1つの症状ですが、あなたはもともと顔色が青白いようです。

Pale skin is another symptom, but you look like you have a naturally pale complexion.
> pale complexion：青白い顔色

☐ あなたが悪性貧血だとすれば、下痢や無気力感はありうる症状です。顔色が悪いのもその症状です。

🍀 If you have pernicious anemia, diarrhea and lethargy are possible symptoms. Pale skin is another symptom.

血液検査

☐ あなたは今までの血液検査で貧血を示唆されたことはありますか。

Have you ever had a blood test that indicated you were anemic?

☐ 治療方針を選ぶ前に、症状のタイプを特定するため網状赤血球数を測りたいと思います。

I'd like to get a reticulocyte count to verify the exact type we're dealing with before we choose a course of treatment for you.

☐ これは、検査室があなたの網状赤血球、すなわち、やや未熟な赤血球を検査するといった単なる血液検査です。

This is just a blood test where the lab will take a look at your reticulocytes, which are slightly immature red blood cells.

☐ 網赤血球数（レチクロ）と呼ばれる、別のタイプの血液検査を行うかもしれません。

I may want to do another type of blood test that we call a "retic count" or a "reticulocyte percent."

2 悪性貧血 ●●● Pernicious Anemia

診断

☐ やはり、あなたは悪性貧血です。あなたの場合は、家族歴が大きな要因であるようです。

As I suspected, you do have pernicious anemia. In your case, family history may play a large part.

☐ あなたの病歴を考えると、一定レベルで低い数値が確認されたら、B12の注射、あるいは内服によるB12の大量摂取を開始することになるでしょう。

Given your background, if we see that certain levels are low, we'll probably just start you on B-12 shots or megadoses of oral B-12.

☐ この種の貧血は腸からビタミンB12を吸収することができないことによるものです。

❂ This type of anemia is about not being able to absorb vitamin B-12 from your intestines.

☐ ビタミンB12は自然に食物からたくさん摂取できます。

It's possible to get a lot of vitamin B-12 naturally from food.

☐ この種の貧血症がベジタリアンに見られることがあるのですが、あなたの場合は十中八九、遺伝によるものと思われます。

We sometimes see this type of anemia in vegetarians; although yours seems most likely a result of genetics.

☐ 治療しないまま放置すると、例えばポリープ、胃がん、脳疾患といった好ましくない病状になる可能性があります。

If left untreated, this condition can lead to polyps, stomach cancer, and brain disease, just to name a few of the possible unpleasant outcomes.

▶ if left untreated：治療しないまま放置すると
　just to name a few：2、3例を挙げると

☐ IF（内因子）が欠乏しているようです。IFは胃が分泌するプロテインで、B12の吸収に必要です。

You seem to have a lack of IF, intrinsic factor. This is a protein that the stomach secretes that is necessary for B-12 absorption.

▶ IF (intrinsic factor)：内因子（胃壁細胞で作られる糖タンパク質）
　secrete：分泌する

Chapter 7 糖尿病代謝内科

1 糖尿病 ●●● Diabetes

糖尿病代謝内科の Dr. Gondo は糖尿病の患者を診察しています。患者は以前の診断結果から、自分の糖尿病についてさほど深刻には考えていないようです。

Dr. I'm looking at the results of your hemoglobin A1c test and you are quite a bit higher than normal. I believe you have diabetes. Have you had a diagnosis of diabetes before?

Pt. No. A couple of years ago, my doctor said I was borderline. So this means I have to stop eating sweets, right?

Dr. Well, I'm not going to recommend sweets, but it's a bit more complicated than that. I want you to do some reading about the glycemic index. Are you familiar with that term?

Pt. I've heard it somewhere, but I'm not sure what it means.

Dr. The glycemic index measures how fast and how much a food raises glucose levels. Choosing to eat foods with lower glycemic index values will help avoid spikes in your blood sugar.

Pt. I think I've also heard people talk about glycemic load.

Dr. I'm glad you brought that up. The glycemic index or GI, as it is called, is very specific as to how quickly a particular carbohydrate breaks down into sugar, but it doesn't take into consideration the amount of carbohydrate in a particular food. So, if you look at glycemic load, the GL, you can get even more information about how that carb will affect your blood sugar.

語句・表現

hemoglobin A1c：
ヘモグロビン・エーワンシー
※赤血球中のヘモグロビンのうちどれくらいの割合が糖と結合しているかを示す検査値。ふだんの血糖値が高い人はHbA1c値が高くなる。

glycemic index (GI)：
グリセミック指数、血糖指数

glucose level：血糖値

glycemic load (GL)：血糖負荷

carbohydrates ＝ carbs：炭水化物

訳

D：あなたのヘモグロビンA1c検査の結果を見ているところですが、正常よりもかなり高いですね。あなたは糖尿病だと思います。今までに、糖尿病だと診断されたことはありますか。

P：いいえ。2、3年前、主治医は私がボーダーライン上だとおっしゃいました。つまりこれは、甘いものを食べるのをやめなければいけないということですよね。

D：まあ、私は甘いものはお勧めしませんが、事はそれ以上に複雑です。あなたには、血糖指数について読んでおいていただきたいです。血糖指数のことはよくご存知ですか。

P：どこかで聞いたことがありますが、どういう意味かはよくわかりません。

D：血糖指数は、食べ物が血糖値をどのくらいの速さで、そしてどのくらい血糖値を上げるかを測定するのです。血糖指数が低い食べ物を選んで摂取すれば、あなたの血糖の急上昇を防ぐ助けとなります。

P：血糖負荷についての話も聞いたことがあるように思います。

D：あなたがその話を持ち出してくれてうれしいです。血糖指数、いわゆるGIは、特定の炭水化物が、どのくらいの速さで糖に分解されるかを明確に示しますが、特定の食物に含まれる炭水化物の量は計算に入っていません。ですので、血糖負荷（GL）を見れば、摂取した炭水化物がどのくらいあなたの血糖に影響を及ぼしているかについて、より多くの情報を得ることができるのです。

雑学
「最初に野菜」の食習慣で1日の血糖値の変動を抑制

　大阪府立大学が、最初に野菜を食べることで血糖値の急激な変化を抑え、糖尿病などの生活習慣病に役立つという研究結果を発表しています。

　血糖の大幅な変動は、脳卒中・心筋梗塞発症につながる細小血管や大血管障害を促すため、食事療法で血糖変動を減らすことが重要です。しかしながら多くの糖尿病の患者さんが「食生活を変更・制限する」ことの難しさに直面しており、「野菜を先に食べる」という簡単な方法で予防・改善が可能になるのは朗報です。

　「よく噛む必要がある」これが野菜を先に食べることのポイントです。野菜には多くの食物繊維が含まれているため「噛まざるを得ない」のです。さらに食物繊維は、腸内での糖分や脂肪分の吸収を抑え、包み込んで排出を促します。また食後の血糖値の上昇を抑える作用があります。

糖尿病代謝内科　使える表現

症状をたずねる

☐ 今までに、糖尿病だと診断されたことはありますか。

❀ Have you had a diagnosis of diabetes before?

☐ ご家族に糖尿病の方はいらっしゃいましたか。

Is there a history of diabetes in your family?

☐ あなたの糖尿病の薬について何か特に問題はありますか。

Have you been having any particular problems with your diabetes medications?

診断

☐ ヘモグロビンA1c検査の結果を見ているところですが正常よりもかなり高いですね。

❀ I'm looking at the results of your hemoglobin A1c test and you are quite a bit higher than normal.

☐ あなたのヘモグロビンA1c検査の数値が先月から上がっていますね。

I see your hemoglobin A1c is up from last month.

☐ あなたの血糖測定器のデータをダウンロードしてみたところ、インスリン注射がうまく行っているようです。

I downloaded the data from your glucometer and it seems that you're doing well with the insulin shots.

☐ 血糖指数は、食べ物が血糖値をどのくらいの速さで、そしてどのくらいの血糖値を上げるかを測定するのです。

❀ The glycemic index measures how fast and how much a food raises glucose levels.

☐ その検査結果はあなたが糖尿病であることを示唆しています。

The tests suggest you have developed diabetes.

☐ あなたのヘモグロビンA1c検査の結果を見たところ、糖尿病ではないと思います。

According to the results of your hemoglobin A1c test, I don't believe you have diabetes.

1 糖尿病 ●●● Diabetes

□ あなたは、実際に近ごろ運動を多くしていらっしゃるので、処方した内服薬はあまり効いていないのではないかと思います。

You've actually been getting more exercise lately, so I'm guessing that the oral medicine we have you on may not be working very well.

処置・処方

□ 日本製で、極めて痛みの少ない特別に細い皮下注射針があります。それを試してみたらどうでしょうか。

There are special small hypodermic needles made in Japan that are quite painless. Why don't you give those a try?

▶ hypodermic needle：皮下注射針

□ **Pt.** その薬はこの病院で、もう入手できますか。

Is that available here yet?

Dr. ご希望でしたら処方できます。しかしながら、私はそうした新しい薬を使ってみることにはちょっと用心しています。

I can prescribe it if you'd like. However, I'm a little leery of trying something so new.

□ この先2ヶ月間、あなたのA1c数値の低下を改善できなかったら、新しい薬を処方するかもしれません。

I may prescribe a new drug if we can't get the A1c lower in the next couple of months.

□ ウェイト・トレーニングをなさってはどうでしょう。

You could consider trying some weight training.

□ 食事の直後に何らかの運動を行うことをお勧めします。

I recommend you get some exercise right after the meal.

□ 適切な食事についての提案をまとめた資料をお渡しします。

I'd like to give you a handout I have on a suggestion for the order in which you eat your meals.

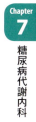

Chapter 8 精神科

1 摂食障害 ●●● Eating Disorders

精神科の Dr. Honda の診察室に摂食障害の娘をもつ母親が訪問しています。Dr. Honda は最近の状況をたずね、アドバイスします。

Dr. How can I help you today, Ms. Peterson?

P.M. (Patient's mother): I appreciate your treating my daughter. She seems a bit calmer lately. I was wondering if there's anything I should be doing differently.

Dr. I know that teenagers sometimes have very busy schedules. Does your daughter eat meals with the family?

P.M. We try to eat together, but, of course it doesn't always work out that way.

Dr. Meal times are the hardest time of the day for teens with eating disorders. If you can make an effort to eat with your daughter and offer balanced meals, that would be very beneficial to her treatment. She needs to feel she's in a comfortable environment and that food is about nourishment, rather than anything else.

Make sure you spend the time enjoying each other's company. You want to discuss neutral topics, rather than focus on food, calories or weight. It would be especially helpful if you can keep her near you and keep the conversation focused on something fun for at least 30 minutes after the meal. This will distract her from purging or feeling guilty about what she's eaten.

P.M. I'll do my best.

語句・表現

eating disorder：摂食障害
nourishment：栄養、滋養物
neutral topic：当たり障りのない話題
distract someone from 〜：（気を散らして）（人）に〜させない
purge：口から胃の内容を放出する

1 摂食障害 ●●● Eating Disorders

訳

D：ピーターソンさん、今日はどうなさいましたか。

PM（患者の母）：娘の治療をしてくださって感謝しております。娘はこの頃、少し落ち着いたようです。私は何か違うことをするべきでしょうか。

D：ティーンエイジャーは非常に忙しいスケジュールを抱えていることが多いものです。お嬢さんはご家族と一緒に食事をしていますか。

PM：一緒に食べるよう心がけていますが、もちろんいつもというわけにはいきません。

D：食事は摂食障害を抱えるティーンエイジャーにとって1日のうちで最も大変な時間です。努めてお嬢さんと一緒に食事を取り、バランスの取れた食事を提供できれば、お嬢さんの治療にとてもプラスになるでしょう。お嬢さんには心地よい環境にいて、他のどんな食事よりも、その食事は栄養があると感じてもらう必要があります。

必ずお互い楽しんで一緒に時間を過ごすようにしてください。食べ物やカロリーや体重のことを重点に置くのではなく、当たり障りのない話をしたいですね。食後、少なくとも30分間お嬢さんをあなたのそばにいさせて、何か楽しいことを中心に会話を続けることができれば、特に役立ちます。こうしたことでお嬢さんを、食べ物の吐き出しや、食べることへの罪悪感から遠ざけるのです。

PM：できるだけやってみます。

雑学
カウンセリング

　摂食障害（過食症・拒食症）の治療は「薬だけでは解決しない」ということが専門家の間でも認識されています。
　英語でのカウンセリングを提供している病院に、「東京カウンセリングサービス」（http://tokyocounseling.com/）があります。
　どの病院でも、一人の患者にかけられる診療時間には限りがあり、ましてや対象となる患者さんが日本語を理解できないということですから、こうした機関の利用は一つの解決策といえるでしょう。ちなみに、病院などでカウンセリングが併設されている場合、保険がきくことはありますが、特別なカウンセリング料が適応される個人の保険等で、カウンセリングを受ける場合を除き、カウンセリングには保険が適用されないのが通例です。

精神科　使える表現

拒食

□ **Dr.** 少しは食べられるようになりましたか。
Are you eating a little better?
Pt. はい、そう思います。少し体重が増えていますが、ゆっくりです。
I think so. I've gained a bit of weight, but it's going slowly.

□ もっと炭水化物を多く食べれば、食習慣を変える手助けになります。
Eating more carbohydrates is helpful for changing your eating habits.
▶ carbohydrates：炭水化物

□ 食事に米やジャガイモやパンを必ず摂取すれば、あなたの食欲を促進する手助けとなるでしょう。
If you make sure to have some rice, potatoes or bread with your meal, that may help stimulate your appetite.

□ 何か人前でくつろいで食べられる食べ物は特にありますか。
Are there some specific foods that you'd be comfortable eating in front of other people?

□ その方策に取り組み、一食も抜かさないようにしてみませんか。
Why don't you just work on that strategy and try not to skip any meals.

過食

□ **Dr.** 何か過食を引き起こすような考え、あるいは行動に思い当たることはありますか。
Can you identify any thoughts or behaviors that trigger binge eating?
Pt. 一人でいるとき、一人ぼっちだと感じるとき、あるいは仕事によるプレッシャーがときどき引き金になるように思います。
I think it happens when I'm alone, feeling lonely, or sometimes the pressure from work triggers it.

治療・助言

□ **Dr.** こうした状況のとき、代わりにできることがありますか。
Can you establish an alternative behavior for these situations?

Pt. そうですね、家にいれば、ギターを弾くことができると思います。
Well, if I'm at home, I guess I can play my guitar.

Dr. それを試していただき、結果を教えてください。
Why don't you give that a try and let me know how it works out.

□ お嬢さんはご家族と一緒に食事をしていますか。
✿ Does your daughter eat meals with the family?

□ 食事は摂食障害を抱えるティーンエイジャーにとって1日のうちで最も大変な時間です。
✿ Meal times are the hardest time of the day for teens with eating disorders.

□ **Dr.** 治療方法のひとつは日記を書くことです。あなたがどう考え、どう感じているかを日々記録できます。
One therapeutic tool is journaling. You can create a diary to write down what you're thinking or feeling.

Pt. どのくらい書く必要がありますか。
How much do I need to write?

Dr. あなたにお任せしますが、衝動脅迫がなくなるまで書き続けるといいでしょう。
That's up to you, but you might want to keep writing until the compulsion passes.

▶ therapeutic tool：治療手段　　journal：日記を書く
You might want to ～．：～するといいでしょう。
compulsion：衝動強迫、脅迫行為　＊本人も無意味な行動だとわかっているのに、止められない衝動。

Chapter 8 精神科

2 うつ病 ●●● Depression

遠い異国に来たことによるホームシックからうつ状態にある患者が、Dr. Hondaの診察を受けに来ています。

Dr. You said that you've been feeling "depressed" for a while. What made you decide to come in? ✼

Pt. My wife pointed out that I used to be much happier. It seems that I lash out at her and I'm always in a bad mood. I think she's right. I was happier before.

Dr. Could you describe the situation to me in a bit more detail?

Pt. Sure. Before I came to Japan I was outgoing and I had lots of friends. These days, I don't seem to be able to make friends and I don't find myself that interested in socializing with the ones I have.

Dr. Do you think you're a little homesick? ✼

Pt. Possibly, but I think it's more than that. I'm here with my family and they all seem to be adjusting fine.

Dr. I understand you've been having trouble sleeping? ✼

Pt. Yes.

Dr. How's your appetite been?

Pt. I don't have much of an appetite these days, actually.

Dr. How much exercise are you getting?

Pt. I've been so tired lately that I haven't felt up to exercising much at all. I don't have a lot of energy. It's almost like I'm in a fog.

Dr. I have a little survey I'd like you to fill out. ✼ Is that all right?

Pt. Sure.

2 うつ病 ●●● Depression

訳

D：あなたは、しばらくの間、気分が「落ち込んだ」状態にあるとのことですね。受診することに決めたきっかけは何でしたか。

P：妻から、私は以前はもっと楽しそうだったと指摘されました。私は妻を厳しく非難し、いつも機嫌が悪いようです。彼女は正しいと思います。以前は気分が明るかったのです。

D：状況をもう少し詳しく説明してもらえますか。

P：はい。日本へ来る前、私は社交的で、たくさんの友だちがいました。近頃は、友だち作りができるようには思えませんし、今の友だちと付き合うことに興味を感じません。

D：少しホームシックだと思いますか。

P：たぶんそうでしょうが、それ以上のことだと思います。ここには家族と一緒に来ていますし、家族はみな、うまく適応しているようです。

D：あなたは睡眠に問題を抱えているのですね。

P：はい。

D：食欲はどうですか。

P：実のところ、この頃あまり食欲がありません。

D：運動はどのくらい行っていますか。

P：最近とても疲れるので、まったく運動する気になりません。あまり体力がありません。まるで霧の中にいるかのようです（途方にくれています）。

D：簡単な調査表に記入していただきたいと思います。よろしいですか。

P：はい。

語句・表現

depressed：精神的に落ち込んだ、うつ状態の

What made you decide to ～？：～することに決めたきっかけは何でしたか。

Chapter 8 精神科

精神科　使える表現

症状・問題をたずねる

☐ あなたは、しばらくの間気分が「落ち込んだ」状態にあるとのことですね。受診することに決めたきっかけは何でしたか。

❋ You said that you've been feeling "depressed" for a while. What made you decide to come in?

☐ 少しホームシックだと思いますか。

❋ Do you think you're a little homesick?

☐ **Dr.** これは最近の問題ですか。
Is this a recent problem?
Pt. はい。数週間前に始まりました。
Yes. It just started a few weeks ago.

☐ **Dr.** 最近この症状を引き起こしただろうと考えられる何かがありましたか。
Has anything happened recently that you think may have caused this?
Pt. 私は少々職場でストレスを受けていますが、それはしょっちゅうあることです。
I'm a little stressed at work, but that's always the case.

☐ 原因となるかもしれない、あなたの生活を変えるような何かに心当たりはありますか。
Can you think of anything that's changed in your life that may be causing it?

☐ 最近どのように感じているかについてもう少し詳しく説明していただけますか。
Could you describe in more detail how you've been feeling lately?

☐ あなたは睡眠に問題を抱えているのですね。

❋ I understand you've been having trouble sleeping?

☐ **Dr.** 睡眠に問題があるとのことですね。
You say you're having trouble sleeping?
Pt. はい。何かそのための薬を先生に処方していただきたいと思いました。
Yes. I was hoping you could prescribe something for it.

2 うつ病 ●●● **Depression**

☐ 簡単な調査表に記入していただきたいと思います。
❀ I have a little survey I'd like you to fill out.

☐ この短い調査に回答していただくことから始めましょう。
Let's start by having you take this short survey.

検査・処方

☐ 血液検査を行い、甲状腺の状態を確認したいと思います。甲状腺機能の低下がうつ病の症状を引き起こすことがあるのです。これは甲状腺機能低下症と呼ばれます。
I want to run a blood test and check out the condition of your thyroid. Sometimes, a low thyroid can cause depression symptoms. It's called hypothyroidism.
▶ thyroid：甲状腺　　hypothyroidism：甲状腺機能低下症

☐ 抗うつ剤を処方しましょう。この薬が（症状の改善に）役に立つかどうかを確かめるため、数週間後に再診していだたきたいと思います。
I'm going to prescribe an antidepressant. I'd like to see you again in a few weeks to see if this is helping.
▶ antidepressant：抗うつ剤

☐ 人によって効き目のある薬は異なりますので、私たちの方針が正しいかどうかを調べたいのです。
Different drugs work better for different people, so I'd like to find out whether or not we're on the right track.
▶ on the right track：正しい方向に向いて

☐ 甲状腺の諸問題に対処し、そのことがうつ病の改善に役立つかどうか確認しましょう。
Let's address the issues with your thyroid and see if that helps with the depression.

☐ 甲状腺機能低下の治療後もうつ状態にあるようなら、抗うつ剤の処方を再検討しましょう。
If you're still depressed after we treat your hypothyroidism, we can revisit the idea of putting you on an antidepressant.
▶ put on 〜：〜を処方する

Chapter 8 精神科

3 双極性障害　Bipolar Disorder

精神科のDr. Hondaはカナダで主治医から双極性障害と診断された患者の日本での治療を行うことになりました。

Dr. You say that your doctor in Canada diagnosed you with bipolar disorder?

Pt. Yes.

Dr. Since I'll be taking over your case, and each case is a little different, I was wondering if you could give me a brief summary of your symptoms.

Pt. Until a year and a half ago, I was what you would have called even-tempered. I didn't get angry easily. Around that time, I developed a short fuse. Everything that didn't go my way was irritating to me. I knew that this kind of behavior was over the top. I tried to monitor myself, but the mood sort of took over, you know what I mean?

Dr. I can imagine.

Pt. After a while, it wasn't just the foul moods. I had these bursts of energy and I wasn't able to sleep. My mind was racing frequently and I realized that I was talking much faster than usual.

Dr. I see.

Pt. Well, this was great, in some ways, because I'm a designer. I was able to create these beautiful sketches. So, to tell the truth, I didn't want it to stop. Unfortunately, after a few days, I'd have to deal with the effects of not enough sleep and I'd start to feel bad.

Dr. I'd like to have you answer a list of questions that you may have answered in your sessions with your doctor back home. The tools I use are based on the U.S. standards from the DSM 5, which I think is fairly standard.

3 双極性障害 ●●● Bipolar Disorder

訳

D：カナダであなたの主治医が双極性障害と診断されたとのことですが。

P：はい。

D：私があなたの症例を引き継ぎますが、個々の症状は少しずつ違うので、あなたの症状の概要を教えていただければと思います。

P：1年半前までは、先生なら、情緒が安定しているとおっしゃっただろう状態でした。私はすぐ怒るようなことはなかったです。その頃、私は癇癪（かんしゃく）を発症しました。私の好きなようにならなかったすべてに、イライラしました。こうした類の言動が度を超えていたことは知っていました。私は自分の行動を監視しようと試みましたが、なんというか、憂うつな気分が優っていました。私の言いたいことがおわかりでしょうか。

D：見当がつきます。

P：しばらくすると、憂うつな気分だけではなったのです。私はこうしたほとばしるエネルギーに満ち、眠ることができませんでした。私は始終あれこれと考えており、気がつくと普段よりもずっと速く話していました。

D：なるほど。

P：まあ、私はデザイナーですから、このことは、ある意味では素晴らしかったのです。短い時間で、これらの美しいスケッチを創り出すことができました。ですから正直なところ、その状態を止めたくありませんでした。残念なことに、数日後には、十分な睡眠をとれなかった影響に対処せざるを得ず、落ち込み始めました。

D：あなたに質問リストに回答していただきたいと思います。質問リストは、治療期間中に、故郷の主治医の先生に回答されたものかもしれませんが。私が使っているツールは、DSM 5（「精神疾患の診断・統計マニュアル」第5版）による米国標準に基づくものでして、私は、それはかなり標準的だと思います。

語句・表現

bipolar disorder：双極性障害
＊以前は躁鬱病（manic depression）と呼ばれていた。
take over ～：～を引き継ぐ
even-tempered：情緒が安定した

short fuse：癇癪（かんしゃく）
go one's way：（人）の好きなようにする
over the top：度を超えて
foul mood：不機嫌、憂うつ

Chapter 8 精神科

精神科　使える表現

症状をたずねる

☐ カナダであなたの主治医が双極性障害と診断されたとのことですが。

❁You say that your doctor in Canada diagnosed you with bipolar disorder?

☐ **Dr.** 何か他に思い出せる症状はありますか。

Are there any other symptoms that you can recall?

Pt. ええと、初期の段階、私はひどい酒飲みでした。私はある種の自己治療を行っているのだと自分に言い聞かせていたのです。たとえ、何杯か酒を飲んだ後に気分がよくなったとしても、私は酒をやめました。今、断酒2年目です。

Well, early on, I was drinking too much alcohol. It's been suggested to me that I was doing some sort of self-medicating. Even though I think I feel better after a couple of drinks, I've quit. I'm two years sober now.

▶ self-medicating：自己治療
＊米国では医師の治療が望ましいのに自力で治そうとするというマイナスイメージで使われることが多い。

▶ ~ years sober：断酒～年目
＊米国の飲酒問題を解決したいと願う相互援助の集まりアルコホーリクス・アノニマス（Alcoholics Anonymous：AA）に加入している人がよく用いる表現。

☐ 個々の症状は少しずつ違うので、あなたの症状の概要を教えていただければと思います。

❁Since each case is a little different, I was wondering if you could give me a brief summary of your symptoms.

☐ **Dr.** あなたが「不機嫌」と呼んでいる状態についてもう少し詳しく説明していただけますか。

Could you describe in more detail what you are calling "foul moods"?

Pt. 何だか、私には心を支配している邪悪な双子がいるかのようでした。そのため私は薬を飲みました。そうすると自分が自分ではないような気もしました。

It was almost as if I had an evil twin that was controlling my mind. So, I took the meds. I didn't feel like me then, either.

▶ foul：不快な、不愉快な
not feel like oneself：自分自身でないような気がする

☐ **Dr.** 薬を飲んだ後はどうでしたか。
How were you after the medication?
Pt. かなり落ち着きました。
I felt much calmer.

診断・処置・処方

☐ 検査の評価に基づき、私はあなたが双極性障害だと思います。
Based on the evaluation, I believe you have bipolar disorder.

☐ 新しい治療法はたくさんあります。たぶん、ブレインフォグを引き起こさないようなものを見つけられるでしょう。
There are lots of new treatments. Maybe we can find something that doesn't cause the brain fog.
▶ brain fog：ブレインフォグ ＊思考に霧がかかったような状態。

☐ 気分を落ち着かせるのに効く薬を処方しましょう。
I'd like to prescribe some medication that I think will help you feel calmer.

☐ 薬の投薬量や考えられる副作用について説明します。
Let me explain the dosage and possible side effects.

雑学
DSM（精神障害／疾患の診断・統計マニュアル）

　米国精神医学会（American Psychiatric Association: APA）が出版するDSM（The Diagnostic and Statistical Manual of Mental Disorders）は、心の健康の「バイブル」とされています。DMSは、多種多様な精神疾患を共通語（英語）で評価した症例モデルのカテゴリー分類体系であり、DSMはその邦訳書において「精神障害／疾患の診断・統計マニュアル」と訳されています。1952年の初版以降、精神医療分野の学会での研究知見に密接に対応し数多くの改訂版が出版されています。
　各改訂版のナンバリングには、初版（DSM-I）以降、ローマ数字が使用されてきましたが、興味深いのは、出版社は、2013年5月出版の最新版には、ローマ数字を使用しないと決定し、DSM-5と表記したことです。これは、大文字のVとの混同を避けるためと思われます。最新版は、初版の8倍の厚さです。

Chapter 9 - リウマチ科

1 関節リウマチ ●●● Rheumatoid Arthritis

リウマチ科の Dr. Iguchi は、長い間リウマチを患っている患者を診察しています。今までかかっていたリウマチ専門医が引退したそうです。

Dr. I understand that your previous rheumatologist has retired and that's why you've come to our hospital. I think the nurse may have mentioned to you that we'd like to take a look at your medical records, if possible.

Pt. Yes. I'll have the other hospital forward them to you.

Dr. I know it's difficult for you to write, so could you give me just a bit of an oral history?

Pt. Sure. The onset of the RA was when I was 27, so I've been dealing with it for more than 35 years. I'm on methotrexate at the moment. Actually, I had a bout with cancer last year and had to go off of the methotrexate for a while. I used prednisone during chemotherapy.

Dr. Were you on other drugs before methotrexate?

Pt. Yes. I was on etanercept before it was approved in Japan. I used to bring it back from the States for personal use. A long time ago, I had treatments with a gold preparation that my Japanese doctor recommended. I've tried various drugs.

Dr. I assume that these therapies began to lose their efficacy after a while.

Pt. Well, there was that and I also had to go off of various treatments because my liver tests were coming back with frighteningly high numbers.

Dr. Of course. A lot of these medications can have a negative effect on your liver.

語句・表現

rheumatologist：リウマチ専門医
medical record：カルテ、医療記録
forward：〜を転送する、送付する
onset：発病
RA：関節リウマチ（Rheumatoid Arthritis の略）
methotrexate：メトトレキサート

1 関節リウマチ ●●● Rheumatoid Arthritis

訳

D：今までかかっていたリウマチ専門医が引退され、あなたは私たちの病院に来られたのですね。できればあなたのカルテの一覧を拝見したいということは、看護師が話したと思います。

P：はい。今まで通った病院に先生宛てにカルテの転送を依頼します。

D：書いていただくのは大変でしょうから、少しだけ病歴を口頭で話してもらえますか。

P：もちろんです。関節リウマチの発病は27歳でしたので、私はこの病気と35年以上取り組んできました。現在は、メトトレキサートを服用しています。実は私は昨年がんで闘病し、しばらくの間メトトレキサートの使用を停止せざるを得ませんでした。化学療法を受ける間はプレドニゾンを使用しました。

D：メトトレキサートの前に別の薬を使っていましたか。

P：はい。エタネルセプトを、それが日本で承認される前から使っていました。かつては個人使用目的でアメリカから持ち帰りました。ずっと前は、日本の主治医が推薦してくれた金製剤を用いた治療を受けていました。私はさまざまな薬を試してきました。

D：これらの治療が、しばらくして効かなくなり始めたようですね。

P：ええと、その通りでしたし、私はさまざまな治療も中止しなくてはなりませんでした。肝臓の検査結果が再び恐ろしいほど高くなったからです。

D：もちろんです。こうした多くの治療はあなたの肝臓に悪影響を与える場合があります。

＊もともと乾癬、がんに用いられていたが、それらの疾患に加え、関節リウマチ、小児リウマチや他の膠原病の治療などに用いられている。

prednisone：プレドニゾン
＊ステロイド系炎症薬。

etanercept：エタネルセプト
＊一般的に関節炎の治療に使われる薬物。がんの治療やがん患者の食欲不振と体重減少に対する治療法の一つとしても研究されている。

gold preparation：金製剤
＊金の有機化合物を原料とする、抗リウマチ薬の一つ。

go off ～：～の使用を中止する

リウマチ科　使える表現

症状をたずねる

☐ 書いていただくのは大変でしょうから、少しだけ病歴を口頭で話してもらえますか。

❋ I know it's difficult for you to write, so could you give me just a bit of an oral history?

☐ **Dr.** どうなさいましたか。

What seems to be the trouble?

Pt. 最近、朝方とてもこわばるのです。

Recently, I've been very stiff in the mornings.

☐ **Dr.** 動き始めると治りますか。

Does it go away after you start moving around?

Pt. 徐々に治りますが、少しは普通に感じるまでに1時間以上かかります。

Eventually, but it takes more than an hour until I feel a little more normal.

▶ go away：（病気・症状が）治る、癒える

☐ **Pt.** かかりつけの医師から先生を紹介されました。最近肘の皮下組織にいくつか腫れ物があることに気がついたからです。

My regular doctor sent me to see you because I've recently noticed some bumps of tissue under the skin on my elbows.

Dr. ちょっと診てみましょう。ああ、腫れ物は堅いですね。

Let's have a look. ... Ah, these bumps are firm.

▶ bump：瘤（こぶ）、腫れ物　　tissue under the skin：皮下組織

☐ メトトレキサートの前に別の薬を使っていましたか。

❋ Were you on other drugs before methotrexate?

☐ まずリウマチ因子を探す簡単な血液検査をしましょう。

Let's first do some simple blood work to look for rheumatoid factor.

▶ blood work：血液検査　　rheumatoid factor：リウマチ因子

1 関節リウマチ ●●● Rheumatoid Arthritis

診断

☐ 残念ながら、私たちは何が関節リウマチの原因なのかよくわかりません。

Unfortunately, we really don't know what causes the RA.

☐ 関節リウマチは免疫システムの障害です。免疫システムが病気と闘うのではなく、自分の身体組織と闘っています。具体的に言うと関節をつなぐ滑膜という厚い膜を攻撃するのです。

RA is an immune system disorder. Instead of the immune system working to fight disease, it is fighting against the body's own tissue. To be more specific, it attacks the synovium, which is a thick membrane that lines your joints.

▶ synovium：滑膜（関節を包む膜のこと）　thick membrane：厚膜
　line the joint：関節をつなぐ

☐ 関節リウマチ患者の約80％は血液中に、私たちがリウマチ因子あるいは略してRF因子と呼んでいる異常な抗体を持っています。

About 80% of rheumatoid arthritis patients have an unusual antibody in their blood that we call rheumatoid factor, or RF for short.

▶ antibody：抗体　rheumatoid factor：リウマチ因子

☐ RF（リウマチ因子）が検査で陰性であっても、他の特別な抗体が陽性となる人がいます。

When someone tests negative for RF, they then sometimes test positive for other special antibodies.

処置・処方

☐ いくつか血液検査をして、数枚Ｘ線写真を撮りましょう。そうすれば症状が把握できます。

Let's run some blood tests and get a few X-rays, so we can see what's going on.

☐ 生物製剤を使っていただきたいと思います。

I want to put you on a biologic.

▶ biologic：生物製剤

☐ 新型の関節リウマチ治療薬です。生物製剤はヒトの遺伝子由来の遺伝子組み換えタンパクです。

It's a new type of medication for RA. Biologics are genetically-engineered proteins that are derived from human genes.

▶ genetically-ngineered protein：遺伝子組み換えタンパク

Chapter 10 一般外科

1 虫垂炎 ●●● Appendicitis

一般外科のDr. Jinkawaは腹部の痛みなど体の不調を訴える患者を診察しています。右下腹部に痛みがあるようです。

CD 2 -19

Dr. What seems to be the trouble today?

Pt. I don't really know. I started out having heartburn. Then, I had this sharp pain near my navel that moved down my abdomen on the right.

Dr. Any nausea?

Pt. Yes, for days as a matter of fact. Last night, I actually threw up. I finally fell asleep, but the pain woke me up. I tried standing up, but that hurt even worse.

Dr. Have you had any trouble passing gas?

Pt. Come to think of it, yes.

Dr. I'd like to take your temperature. … As I suspected, you have a low-grade fever. Tell me, did it hurt worse when I pushed down or when I let go?

Pt. When you let go.

Dr. Ah, rebound tenderness leads me to suspect appendicitis. Actually, you're exhibiting all the classic signs of appendicitis. I'd like to have you meet with the surgeon. It's better to do appendectomies as soon as possible.

Pt. I need surgery?

Dr. Yes, I'm afraid so. I think the surgeon will opt to do this laparoscopically, so there will be a shorter recovery period.

語句・表現

heartburn：胸焼け
navel：へそ
abdomen：腹部
nausea：吐き気
pass gas：おならをする

let go：離す
rebound tenderness：反跳痛
appendicitis：虫垂炎
appendectomy：虫垂切除術
laparoscopically：腹腔鏡下で

1 虫垂炎 ●●● Appendicitis

訳

D：今日はどうなさいましたか。

P：よくわからないのです。胸焼けがし始めました。その後、この鋭い痛みをへその近くに感じ、それが腹部の右側の方へと移動しました。

D：吐き気はどうですか。

P：はい、実際のところ何日間も。昨晩は、実は吐きました。私はようやく眠りにつきましたが、痛くて目が覚めました。私は立ち上がろうとしましたが、痛みがますます悪化しました。

D：おならが出にくかったりしましたか。

P：そう言われれば、はい、そうでした。

D：熱を測らせてください。思った通り、微熱がありますね。私が手で押したときか、手を離したときか、より痛みが増した方を教えてください。

P：先生が手を離したときです。

D：ああ、反跳痛がありますので、虫垂炎の疑いがあります。実際、典型的な虫垂炎の兆候がすべて見られます。外科医を紹介しましょう。虫垂切除手術をできるだけ早く受けた方がいいですよ。

P：手術が必要なのですか。

D：はい、残念ながら。外科医は手術を腹腔鏡で行うと思いますので、回復にかかる期間は早まるでしょう。

表現のポイント

★ **appendix と appendicitis**
虫垂（appendix）に起こる炎症は appendicitis と言います。(-itis) を付けると炎症を表します。

★ **rebound tenderness（反跳痛）**
盲腸の初期症状では、腹痛を伴いますが、反跳痛と呼ばれる痛みが出ることがあります。反跳痛は、腹部を圧迫して離したときの痛みを示します。医師は、押し下げたとき（push down）の痛み「圧痛」と、離したとき（let go）の痛み「反跳痛」を観察します。

Chapter 10 一般外科

●●● 一般外科　使える表現

症状をたずねる

- [ ] **Dr.** 痛みに最初に気付いたのはいつですか。
  When did you first notice your pain?
  > **Pt.** 1時間前から急に痛みが強くなりましたが、昨日から吐き気がして、その度に胃の辺りが痛みます。
  > It got really bad an hour ago, but I've been nauseated since yesterday, and whenever I feel nauseous, it hurts around my stomach.

- [ ] おならが出にくかったりしましたか。
- ❈ Have you had any trouble passing gas?

診察

- [ ] **Dr.** 痛む所を見せていただけますか。
  Can you show me where the pain is?
  Pt. ここです。
  Right here.
  Dr. ああ、へその近くですね。あおむけに寝ていただけますか。
  Ah, it's close to your belly button. I'd like you to lie down on your back.

- [ ] さて、これから強めに押して、痛むかどうか聞いていきますね。
  Now, I'm going to press rather hard and ask you if it hurts.

- [ ] ここの部分、前腕の内側の2本の腱の間を、手首から約指3本分下のところで押してください。そこは吐き気を和らげるツボです。
  I want you to press here, between the two tendons inside your forearm, about three fingers down from your wrist. It's an acupressure point that helps with nausea.
  ▶ forearm：前腕（肘から手首までの部分）　　acupressure point：ツボ

- [ ] この検査は「ロブシング徴候」と呼ばれており、最初にその手法を確認したデンマーク人の外科医にちなんで名付けられました。
  This test is called "Rovsing's sign," it's named after the Danish surgeon who first identified the technique.

1 虫垂炎 ●●● Appendicitis

▶ Rovsing's sign：ロブシング徴候
＊腹膜炎の際に、腹壁を強く圧迫し、左下腹部を圧迫すると右下腹部の痛みが増強する徴候。

☐ もう2、3種類の検査をやってみます。よい結果が出たら、抗生物質を1コース試しましょう。

I'm going to try a few more tests. If we get positive results, we'll put you on a course of antibiotics.

☐ 抗生物質の投与を1ラウンド終えたら、また診察させてください。

I'd like to see you again after you finish a round of antibiotics.

▶ antibiotics：抗生物質
course / round：治療単位。どちらかというと、courseの方が正式な言い方で、roundの方がくだけた言い方。

診断

☐ 反跳痛がありますので、虫垂炎の疑いがあります。典型的な虫垂炎の兆候がすべて見られます。

✿ Rebound tenderness leads me to suspect appendicitis. You're exhibiting all the classic signs of appendicitis.

☐ 急性虫垂炎かもしれません。白血球数を検査したいと思います。

You may have acute appendicitis. I'd like to check your white blood cell count.

▶ acute appendicitis：急性虫垂炎

☐ 看護師に車椅子を持ってきてもらって、緊急治療室（ER）にお連れします。

I'll have the nurse get a wheelchair to take you to the ER.

☐ 虫垂切除手術をできるだけ早く受けた方がいいですよ。

✿ It's better to do appendectomies as soon as possible.

☐ 虫垂切除術の日時を決める必要があります。

We need to think about scheduling you for an appendectomy.

☐ 外科医は手術を腹腔鏡で行うと思いますので、回復にかかる期間は早まるでしょう。

✿ I think the surgeon will opt to do this laparoscopically, so there will be a shorter recovery period.

Chapter 10 一般外科

2 胆石 ... Gallstones

Dr. Jinkawaの診察室を訪れた患者には、胸骨のすぐ下に痛みがあります。
非常に多忙な患者のようですが、Dr. Jinkawaのアドバイスは…。

Dr. Could you describe the pain?

Pt. Well, until yesterday it would come and go. I'd get these sudden pains right under my breastbone and then I'd feel better. But today, I felt like I just couldn't get comfortable.

Dr. I'd like to do an ultrasound of your abdomen and get a CT scan.

Pt. What do you think this is?

Dr. I believe there's a high likelihood that you have gallstones. I don't know you well, but I think you look a little jaundiced. I want to run some blood tests to make sure we aren't dealing with infection or other associated complications.

Pt. Oh, all right. You have medicine to dissolve them, right?

Dr. The medicine we have doesn't usually work right away, so you may still have the pain for quite a while, which is rarely a good idea. Besides, once you develop gallstones they're very likely to return. The usual treatment for this condition is surgery.

Pt. Wow. I'm really busy at work now. I can't take a lot of time off …

Dr. Well, you aren't going to be able to work in constant pain, either. You don't need to worry about a long recovery period. These days, this is usually a laparoscopic procedure. We insert a tiny video camera along with some special surgical tools through four small incisions and we get a good view of your gallbladder on the screen and remove it. The hospital stay for this is quite short. Most of my patients go back to work in a week.

2 胆石 ●●● Gallstones

訳

D：痛みについてご説明いただけますか。

P：はい、昨日までは現れたり消えたりしていました。こうした突然の痛みを胸骨のすぐ下に感じ、それから具合がよくなったのです。ところが今日はよくならないようです。

D：腹部の超音波とCTスキャンを行いたいと思います。

P：何の病気だとお考えですか。

D：胆石である可能性が高いと思います。あなたのことはよく存じ上げませんが、少し黄疸があるように見えます。感染症あるいはその他の合併症を伴っていないか確認するために、いくつか血液検査を行いたいと思います。

P：ああ、わかりました。それらを溶かす薬があるのですよね。

D：処方する薬は通常、直ちに効くわけではないので、まだ当分は痛みがあるかもしれません。薬はうまくいかないことが多いのです。その上、胆石は発症すると、（薬を使っても）再発する可能性が極めて高いのです。この症状について治療は通常手術です。

P：うわっ、私は今とても仕事が忙しいのです。長く休むことはできません。

D：あの、絶えず続く痛みを抱えていては働くこともできませんよ。回復にかかる期間のことは心配する必要はありません。近年はたいてい腹腔鏡による手術です。特別な手術ツールのついた極めて小さなビデオカメラを4つの小さな切開部から挿入し、画面上に胆嚢がよく見えるようにして、それを切除します。この手術による入院はとても短期間です。私の患者のほとんどは1週間で仕事に戻ります。

語句・表現

breastbone：胸骨
abdomen：腹部
jaundiced：黄疸にかかった
complications：合併症
for quite a while：かなり長い時間
laparoscopic：腹腔鏡下の
incision：切開
gallbladder：胆嚢（のう）

Chapter 10 一般外科

●●● 一般外科　使える表現

診察

☐ あなたは6ヶ月前に胆嚢摘除をされたのですね。

You had a cholecystectomy six months ago.
▶ cholecystectomy：胆嚢摘除

☐ あなたはどういった食事療法をなさっていますか。

What's your diet like?

☐ 乳製品、油っこい料理、甘すぎる食べ物、それからカフェインを避けることをお勧めします。

I suggest that you avoid dairy products, greasy food, excessively sweet food and caffeine.
▶ greasy food：油っこい料理、脂肪分の多い料理

☐ 少し黄疸があるように見えます。感染症あるいはその他の合併症を伴っていないか確認するために、いくつか血液検査を行いたいと思います。

❀**I think you look a little jaundiced. I want to run some blood tests to make sure we aren't dealing with infection or other associated complications.**

☐ 切開した部分を診たいと思います。(中断) はい、懸念したとおりです。切開部分が感染しています。抗生物質を処方しましょう。

I'd like to take a look at your incision. (pause) Yes, just as I suspected. The incision is infected. I'm putting you on antibiotics.

☐ 感染症は常に慎重に扱うべきですが、これは表在感染だと思いますので、抗生物質で症状に対応できるでしょう。

Infections should always be treated seriously, but I believe this is a superficial infection and the antibiotics should take care of the issue.
▶ superficial infection：表在感染

手術の説明

☐ この症状について治療は通常手術です。

❀**The usual treatment for this condition is surgery.**

2 胆石 ●●● Gallstones

- 近年はたいてい腹腔鏡による手術です。
- ❈ These days, this is mostly a laparoscopic procedure.

- 特別な手術ツールのついた極めて小さなビデオカメラを4つの小さな切開部から挿入し、画面上に胆嚢がよく見えるようにして、それを切除します。
- ❈ We insert a tiny video camera along with some special surgical tools through four small incisions and we get a good view of your gallbladder on the screen and remove it.

- 手術後、ほとんどの人は比較的すぐに下痢が止まりますが、下痢が続く患者もいます。
- The diarrhea stops relatively soon after surgery for most people, but there are patients that continue to have trouble with it.

手術前の注意

- 手術前日は、クリアリキッド（水やお茶、清涼飲料水など）以外は口にしないでください。
- You'll need to drink clear liquids only on the day before the surgery.

- これはあなたのための情報シートで、手術前にすべきことについてすべて説明されています。
- This is an information sheet for you that explains everything else you'll need to do prior to the operation.

- その薬は手術の5日前に中止してください。
- I want you to stop that five days before surgery.

- アスピリンやその他の薬、あるいはここに掲載されているサプリメントは服用しないでください。
- Don't take any aspirin or any of the other drugs or supplements that are listed here.

- 夜の12時以降は何も飲まないでください。日中は、澄んだスープやお茶の類は口にして結構です。
- Don't drink anything after midnight. During the day you can have clear soup, tea and that sort of thing.

- 手術について何か他に質問はありますか。
- Do you have any other questions about the surgery?

Chapter 10 一般外科

3　腰痛・背痛　●●● Backache

一般外科のDr. Jinkawaは、今日は背中に痛みを訴える患者を診察しています。

Pt. I've got a terrible backache. At first, I thought I'd just slept funny, but it doesn't want to go away.

Dr. Can you show me where it hurts?

Pt. Right here.

Dr. Does it hurt if I press here?

Pt. A little, but not as much.

Dr. Does coughing or sneezing make it worse?

Pt. Yes.

Dr. Do you have any other symptoms?

Pt. Nothing comes to mind.

Dr. Have you been taking anything for the pain?

Pt. Just some ibuprofen that I brought with me to Japan.

Dr. This seems like a muscle issue to me. I'd like to prescribe a muscle relaxant. I'm only going to give you a two-week dose. I'd also like to give you something for the pain.

Pt. So the pain will be gone in two weeks?

Dr. We can hope so, but the reason that the dosage is done that way is that muscle relaxers lose the ability to be effective on the actual muscles after roughly two weeks. The majority of back pain goes away in that period of time. I'll give you the prescription for the muscle relaxer and ask you to come back and see me when you run out of the medicine. I'd like to ask you not to drive for the next two weeks, as the medicine will make you drowsy. You may also feel some muscle weakness.

3 腰痛・背痛 ●●● Backache

訳

P：ひどく腰が痛みます。最初はただ寝違えたのだと思いましたが、痛みが引きません。

D：どこが痛むか見せていただけますか。

P：ちょうどここです。

D：ここを押すと痛みますか。

P：少し痛みますが、それほどではありません。

D：咳やくしゃみで痛みがひどくなりますか。

P：はい。

D：他に症状はありますか。

P：何も思いつきません。

D：痛みのために何か薬を飲んでいますか。

P：日本へ持参したイブプロフェンだけです。

D：この症状は筋肉のもののようです。筋弛緩剤を処方しましょう。2週間分だけお渡しします。痛みを抑えるものも処方しましょう。

P：では痛みは2週間でなくなると。

D：そう見込めますが、投薬の量を2週間にした理由は、筋弛緩剤が、実際に筋肉への効能を失うのがおおよそ2週間後だからです。腰痛の大多数は2週間でなくなります。筋弛緩剤の処方箋をお渡ししますので、薬が切れる頃に再診してください。薬のために眠くなることもありますので、これから2週間は運転をしないようお願いします。筋力の低下も感じるかもしれません。

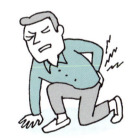

語句・表現

ibuprofen：イブプロフェン　＊非ステロイド系解熱鎮痛、抗炎症薬

muscle relaxant [relaxer]：筋弛緩剤

drowsy：眠気を誘う

Chapter 10 一般外科

●●● 一般外科　使える表現

症状をたずねる

- [ ] **Dr.** どうなさいましたか。
  What seems to be the problem?
  Pt. 首の筋を違えました。
  I have a crick in my neck.

- [ ] **Dr.** 痛みについて話していただけますか。
  Could you describe your pain for me?
  Pt. ここ１週間、肩（首）が凝っています。　首の痛みは特に夜になるとひどいのです。
  I've had a stiff neck for the past week. The pain in my neck is especially bad at night.

- [ ] **Dr.** 痛みについて教えてください。
  Tell me about the pain, please.
  Pt. 背面が始終痛み、時にはこの刺すような痛みは足にまで達します。それ以外の時は、足はしびれたような感じです。
  My back hurts most of the time and sometimes I get this shooting pain down my leg. Other times, my leg just feels kind of numb.
  ▶ shooting pain：刺痛、電撃痛

- [ ] **Dr.** どのような痛みか表していただけますか。
  How would you describe the pain?
  Pt. 腰がいつも痛むのですが、時には首も痛みます。
  I mostly have a persistent pain in my tailbone, but sometimes my neck hurts, too.
  ▶ tailbone：尾骨　＊口語では「腰」を意味する。

- [ ] **Dr.** この症状は今までに経験されましたか。
  Have you ever had this before?
  Pt. 数ヶ月前に何かこのようなことがありましたが、症状は消えました。
  I had something like it a few months ago, but it went away.

- [ ] 座ったり、立ったり、横になると痛みは改善しますか、悪化しますか。
  Is it better or worse if you're sitting, or standing, or lying down?

3 腰痛・背痛 ●●● **Backache**

☐ 両下肢に脱力感はありますか。
Do you have any weakness in your legs?

☐ 痛みのために何か薬を飲んでいますか。
✢ Have you been taking anything for the pain?

診断・処方

☐ この症状は筋肉のもののようです。筋弛緩剤を処方しましょう。
✢ This seems like a muscle issue to me. I'd like to prescribe a muscle relaxant.

☐ 薬のために眠くなることもありますので、これから２週間は運転をしないようお願いします。
✢ I'd like to ask you not to drive for the next two weeks, as the medicine will make you drowsy.

☐ これを服用している間は、お酒を飲まないでください。
Don't drink alcohol while you're taking this.

☐ あなたの腰痛は骨の突起によるものだと思われます。
The pain in your back is most likely being caused by bone spurs.
  ▶ bone spur：骨の突起

☐ 狭窄症かもしれません。狭窄とは脊椎の間の隙間が狭くなることです。
You're probably experiencing stenosis, which is a narrowing of the open spaces within your spine.
  ▶ stenosis：狭窄症

表現のポイント

stiff shoulder（肩凝り）と **stiff neck**（首凝り）
技術的に見て、腕を上げることができない状態が stiff shoulder、頭を左右に動かせない状態が stiff neck です。stiff shoulder（肩凝り）は日本でよく用いられる首や肩の痛みの総称表現です。日本では「肩が凝る」とは言いますが、「首が凝る」とはあまり言いません。一方 still neck は英語で非常に一般的に用いられます。実際にウェブ検索をすると圧倒的に stiff neck の方が多くヒットします。shoulder（肩）と neck（首）――同じ痛みでも、言語によって表現の仕方に違いがあるのは興味深いことです。

Chapter 11 - 整形外科

1 捻挫・骨折 ●●● Sprains/Fractures

整形外科の Dr. Kato の診察室では、足をくじいた若い患者に「RICE」というアドバイスをしています。それはいったい何でしょうか。 CD2-22

Dr. What seems to be the trouble?

Pt. I twisted my ankle. It hurts when I put weight on it.

Dr. Is this tender?

Pt. Yes, but not so bad.

Dr. It's a bit swollen, but there's no discoloration. When did this happen?

Pt. Last night. I put ice on it several times.

Dr. I suspect it's a mild sprain. I think we can just wrap it with an Ace bandage and have you stay off of it for a while. This is what we call a Grade 1 Sprain and we recommend "RICE." RICE stands for: Rest, Ice, Compression and Elevation. So, try to limit your walking as much as possible. Alternate wrapping your ankle with the Ace bandage and putting ice on it. Leave the ice packs on for 15 to 20 minutes. Wrap the Ace bandage from the base of your toes to just above your ankle joint. Also, keep your foot elevated, preferably above your heart, as often as possible.

Pt. I'll do my best to rest, but I have a couple of midterm tests this week. I can't stay off of it every day … What should I do?

Dr. Let's not risk making it worse. I think we need to put you on crutches for the next ten days or so. I'll call in my nurse and she'll set you up with a pair.

表現のポイント

Ace bandage（エースバンドエイド）

Aceは包帯の商標ですが、米国では、ACEタイプの包帯全般を示す単語になっています。これは化学調味料の Ajinomoto の商標名が使われているのと同様で、こうした言い回しには、Kleenex ＝ ティッシュ全般、Jell-O ＝ ゼリーのデザート全般、saran wrap ＝ 透明なプラスチック包装などがあります。

1 捻挫・骨折 ●●● Sprains/Fractures

訳

D：どうなさいましたか。

P：足をくじいたのです。体重をかけると足首が痛みます。

D：これは触ると痛みますか。

P：はい、でもそれほど痛くはありません。

D：少し腫れていますが変色はしていませんね。いつくじいたのですか。

P：昨夜です。何度か氷を上にあてました。

D：軽い捻挫だと思います。患部に伸縮性のある包帯を巻くだけにして、しばらく動かさないでそのままにしておきましょう。これはグレード1の捻挫と呼んでいるもので、「RICE」をお勧めします。Rest（安静）、Ice（冷却）、Compression（圧迫、固定）、Elevation（挙上）の略語です。ですので、できるだけ歩き回らないようにして、繰り返し患部を包帯で巻いて氷をあててください。氷は15分から20分あてておいてください。包帯は足指の付け根から足首の関節のま上まで巻いてください。また、できるだけ心臓より高いところに足を持ち上げてください。

P：できるだけ休息を取りますが、今週はいくつか中間テストがあるのです。毎日脚を使わないわけにはいきません。どうしたらいいでしょうか。

D：悪化させないようにしましょう。これから10日間ほど、松葉杖を使ってもらったほうがいいでしょう。看護師を呼んで、1脚用意させましょう。

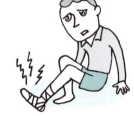

語句・表現

tender：圧痛のある、触ると痛い
swollen：腫れた
discoloration：変色
stay off：～を使わない（動かさない）ようにする
compression：固定
＊compressionは「圧縮（圧搾・圧迫）すること」で、ここでは患部をしっかり巻いて動かないようにするという意味で使われている。
elevate：～を持ち上げる
make ～ worse：～を悪化させる
crutch (crutches)：松葉杖
＊松葉杖は左右2本で使うことが多いので、複数を使うことが多い。

Chapter 11 整形外科

> ●●● **整形外科　使える表現**

症状をたずねる

- **Dr.** どうなさいましたか。
  - What seems to be the trouble?
  - **Pt.** 足をくじいたのです。
  - I twisted my ankle. / I messed up my ankle.

- **Dr.** なぜ足全体があざだらけなのですか。
  - Why's your leg all black and blue?
  - **Pt.** つまずいて転びました。
  - I tripped and fell.
    - ▶ (be) black and blue：（体の部分が）あざだらけである　　trip：つまずく

- **Dr.** 腕をどうなさったのですか。
  - What did you do to your arm?
  - **Pt.** 氷の上で滑って転びました。
  - I slipped and fell on the ice.

- **Dr.** その目の黒あざはどうなさいましたか。
  - How did you get that black eye?
    - ▶ black eye：（目のまわりの）青あざ、黒あざ
    - ＊目のまわり以外の体のあざについては、black and blue を使います。
  - **Pt.** バスで正面の男性がレインコートを着ようとして、私の目を強打したのです。
  - The guy in front of me on the bus went to put on his raincoat and knocked me right in the eye.

診察

- 触ると痛みますか。
- Is this tender?

- 軽い捻挫だと思います。患部に伸縮性のある包帯を巻くだけにして、しばらく動かさないでそのままにしておきましょう。
- I suspect it's a mild sprain. I think we can just wrap it with an Ace bandage and have you stay off of it for a while.

- レントゲンの検査結果は右のくるぶしに細かいひびが入っていることを示しています。
- The X-ray shows a hairline fracture in your right ankle.

1 捻挫・骨折 ●●● Sprains / Fractures

> hairline fracture：（髪の毛のような）細いひび

☐ 検査でははっきりしませんでしたが、レントゲン写真から手首の骨折が明らかです。

I wasn't sure from the examination, but the X-ray reveals that you've actually broken your wrist.

処置・処方

☐ 悪化させないようにしましょう。これから10日間ほど、松葉杖を使ってもらったほうがいいでしょう。

✿ Let's not risk making it worse. I think we need to put you on crutches for the next ten days or so.

☐ エアキャスト®を装着していただきたいと思います。この装具で痛みが軽減しますし、骨折も快方に向かい始めます。

I'd like to put you in an Aircast®. It should relieve the pain and start to heal the fracture, as well.

> Aircast®：エアキャスト（歩行用装具）
> ＊商標を使わないときにはwalking bootといった言い方を使います。

☐ ひどい足首の捻挫用に特別に設計されたウォーキングブーツを着用していただきたいと思います。

I'd like you to wear a walking boot specifically designed for severe ankle sprains.

☐ これから数週間は患部に何の負荷もかけないようにすべきです。

You shouldn't put any weight on it for the next few weeks.

☐ 前回診察したときよりも明らかに悪化しています。膝の人工関節置換手術をお勧めします。

This is definitely worse than the last time I saw you. I'm going to recommend knee replacement surgery.

> knee replacement surgery：膝の人工関節置換手術

☐ 関節のことが気がかりです。リウマチ専門医を紹介したいと思います。

I'm concerned about your joints. I'd like to send you to a rheumatologist.

> rheumatologist：リウマチ専門医

Chapter 11 - 整形外科

2 傷 ... Wounds

Dr. Kato の診察室に父親に付き添われてやってきたのは3歳の男の子です。男の子は頭から出血しています。

CD 2 -23

Dr. Okay, let's sit him up over here. How did he cut his head like this?

P.F. (Patient's father): He was standing up on the sofa playing with his toy soldiers and he fell and hit his head on the coffee table.

Dr. How long ago was this?

P.F. About half an hour ago. We live close by, so I didn't call an ambulance, I just put him in the car and got here as fast as I could. His head was bleeding like crazy.

Dr. It's kind of deep. Can you keep holding that towel on it and applying pressure?

P.F. Sure.

Dr. Ah … Did he lose consciousness or fall asleep at any time?

P.F. No. Of course he was crying at first, but he calmed right down. Actually, he seemed oddly calm.

Dr. I'm sure he's experiencing some shock. We're going to need to give him a few stitches. I think we can use a local anesthetic, so we don't have to move him to an operating room.

P.F. Is he going to have a bad scar?

Dr. I doubt it. His hair should cover it.

語句・表現

bleed like crazy：ひどく出血する
apply pressure：圧迫する
lose consciousness：意識を失う
right down：全く、徹底的に
seem oddly calm：奇妙なほど落ち着いて見える

stitch：（針の）ひと縫
local anesthetic：局所麻酔薬、
scar：傷跡
I doubt it.：私はそうは思いません。さあどうでしょうね。

2 傷 ●●● Wounds

訳

D： では、こちらに息子さんを座らせてください。どうやってこのように頭に切り傷を負ったのですか。

PF（患者の父）： 息子はおもちゃの兵隊で遊びながらソファの上に立っていて、倒れてコーヒーテーブルに頭をぶつけました。

D： どのくらい前にこうなったのですか。

PF： 30分ほど前です。近所に住んでいますので、救急車は呼ばず、息子を車に乗せてできる限り早くここに参りました。頭からものすごく出血していました。

D： ちょっと深いですね。（傷の上を）そのタオルで押さえて圧迫してもらえますか。

PF： わかりました。

D： あ、息子さんはいずれかの時点で意識を失ったり寝入ったりしましたか。

PF： いいえ。もちろん最初は泣きましたが、まったく落ち着いていました。実は奇妙なほど落ち着いて見えました。

D： 息子さんは何らかのショックを経験しているのは確かです。数針縫う必要があります。局所麻酔薬が使えると思うので、手術室に息子さんを移す必要はありません。

PF： ひどい傷跡になりますか。

D： そうは思いません。髪の毛で隠れますよ。

表現のポイント

stitches と staples

stitches と staples は傷口をふさぐ上での代表的な方法です。傷の深さ、状態、傷を負った場所、患者の体調などに応じて方法が選択されますが、それほど深くないような頭部の傷なら staples（ホッチキス［正式にはスキンステープラー］）が、骨や神経に達しているような深い傷や膝、肘、指などのよく動かす部分、顔などの傷を目立たせたくない部分などは stitches（糸で縫合）がよく用いられます。

●●● 整形外科　使える表現

症状をたずねる

- **Dr.** どうなさいましたか。
  What seems to be the trouble?
- **Pt.** タマネギを切っていて包丁がすべりました。
  I was chopping onions and my knife slipped.
- **Dr.** 非常にスパッと切れた切り口です。看護師に患部を消毒して、バタフライ・バンドエイドを貼らせます。今日は、縫合の必要はありません。
  It's a very clean cut. I'll have the nurse disinfect it and apply a butterfly bandage. There's no need for stitches today.
  - ▶ clean cut：スパッと切れた切り口
    butterfly bandage：バタフライ・バンドエイド
    ＊裂口が開かないように留めるバンドエイド。

- どうやってこのように頭に切り傷を負ったのですか。
- How did he get this cut on his head?

- 破傷風の注射をしたのはいつが最後ですか。
  When's the last time you had a tetanus shot?

- 彼はいずれかの時点で意識を失ったり寝入ったりしましたか。
- Did he lose consciousness or fall asleep at any time?

処置・処方

- 傷口がギザギザなので、感染しやすいため縫合したいと思います。
  Because this cut has jagged edges, I'd like to sew it up.
  - ▶ jagged edge：（ガラスの破片などの）ギザギザになった縁

- かなり短いのですが、比較的深い裂傷です。だから感染症を避けるよう、縫合すべきですね。
  It's a fairly short, but relatively deep laceration. So, we should suture it to avoid infection.
  - ▶ laceration：裂傷

- 傷口が感染しないように、患部を清潔に保つよう気をつけてください。
  Be careful to keep the area clean so the wound doesn't become infected.

2　傷　Wounds

☐ この傷は20mm以上の深さのようです。

It seems that this wound is deeper than 20mm.

☐ 傷の感染を防ぐため抗生物質を処方しましょう。

I'm going to prescribe antibiotics to stave off possible wound infection.

☐ 素早く傷口を閉じる必要があったので、ホッチキスを使いました。

We've used staples because we needed to close up the wound quickly.

☐ 軟膏は患部を清潔に湿り気を保つのですが、塗りすぎると皮膚がふやけます。乾燥させておく方がよいと思います。

Ointments keep things clean and moist, but too much ointment can macerate the skin. I prefer to leave it dry.
　▶ macerate：〜をやわらかくする、ふやけさせる

☐ すぐに破傷風の注射をしましょう。

Let's get you a tetanus shot right away.
　▶ tetanus shot：破傷風の予防注射

再診について

☐ これは溶ける縫合糸です。悪化しない限りは再来される必要はありません。

These are dissolvable stitches. There's no need to come back unless it gets worse.
　▶ dissolvable stitch：溶ける縫合糸

☐ 経過を見せに8、9日後にいらしてください。

Come back in eight or nine days for us to take a look.

☐ その時までに適切に治癒していたらホッチキスを外しますし、まだならあと4、5日待ちます。

If it's properly healed by then, we'll remove the staples, if not, we may wait another four or five days.

☐ 受付で予約を取り、10〜12日後に抜糸をしに来てください。

Go ahead and make an appointment with the receptionist to come and have the stitches removed in 10 to 12 days.

Chapter 11 - 整形外科

3 ヘルニア ●●● Hernia

Dr. Katoの元に最近日本に引っ越してきた患者がやって来ました。鼠径（そけい）部の圧迫感を訴えています。

Dr. You say that you feel pressure in your groin?

Pt. Yes. I sometimes have pain, as well.

Dr. I see. Have you done any heavy lifting?

Pt. Well, I did a lot of lifting when we packed up to move to Japan.

Dr. How long have you had this cough?

Pt. I've been coughing a lot for the past few weeks. I think I've had a bit of a cold.

Dr. Are you a smoker?

Pt. Yes.

Dr. That could also account for some of your coughing. Have you ever been diagnosed with a hernia?

Pt. No, not that I can recall.

Dr. You seem to display all the classic symptoms of an inguinal hernia.

Pt. So it happened when I picked up a box or something?

Dr. It's hard to say, but that could've been the trigger. This happens when there's a weakness in the muscle of your abdominal wall. Chronic coughing from smoking is sometimes the culprit. Your hernia is quite small, actually. This makes me want to take a "wait and see" approach. We can set up regular appointments and watch it. The other alternative is surgery.

Pt. I'd like to avoid surgery. The pain is sometimes pretty annoying, though.

Dr. I can prescribe mild painkillers.

3 ヘルニア ●●● Hernia

訳

D：鼠径（そけい）部に圧迫感があるとのことですね。

P：はい。時々痛みもあります。

D：なるほど。何か重いものを持ち上げましたか。

P：あの、私は日本へ引っ越すために荷造りをする際、たくさん持ち上げました。

D：この咳はいつからありますか。

P：ここ数週間、すごく咳が出ます。ちょっと風邪をひいていたのだと思います。

D：タバコをお吸いになりますか。

P：はい。

D：タバコはあなたの咳の主な原因の一部となり得ます。ヘルニアと診断されたことはありますか。

P：いいえ、そう言われたことはなかったと思います。

D：鼠径ヘルニアの典型的な症状がすべて見られるようです。

P：それでその症状は箱やら何やらを持ち上げて起きたのでしょうか。

D：そうとは言いにくいのですが、そのことが引き金となった可能性があります。これは腹部の壁の筋肉が弱いと起こるのです。喫煙による慢性咳嗽（がいそう）は問題の発端となることがあります。あなたのヘルニアは実際には非常に小さいものです。こうした症状の場合、私は「経過観察」のアプローチを取りたいと思います。定期的に診断して、様子を見ます。これに代わる方法は手術ですが。

P：手術は避けたいと思います。痛みにはとても悩まされることがあるのですが。

D：穏やかな痛み止めを処方できます。

語句・表現

groin：鼠径（そけい）部（股の付け根）
inguinal hernia：鼠径ヘルニア
hard to say：言い難い
abdominal wall：腹部の壁

chronic coughing：慢性咳嗽（がいそう）
culprit：問題の発端
wait and see：経過観察

Chapter 11 - 整形外科

整形外科　使える表現

症状をたずねる

☐ 鼠径（そけい）部に圧迫感があるとのことですね。
❋ You say that you feel pressure in your groin?

☐ 何か重いものを持ち上げましたか。
❋ Have you done any heavy lifting?

☐ この咳はいつからありますか。
❋ How long have you had this cough?

☐ ヘルニアと診断されたことはありますか。
❋ Have you ever been diagnosed with a hernia?

診断

☐ あなたには鼠径ヘルニアの典型的な症状がすべて見られるようです。
❋ You seem to display all the classic symptoms of an inguinal hernia.

☐ **Pt.** 私が重い箱を持ち上げたときに起こったのでしょうか。
　　Did it happen when I picked up a heavy box?
　Dr. そうとは言いにくいですが、それが引き金となった可能性があります。
❋ It's hard to say, but doing that could have been the trigger.

☐ この病状は、腸への血流を遮断する絞扼性（こうやくせい）ヘルニアを引き起こす可能性があります。
This condition can lead to a strangulated hernia, which will cut off the blood supply to your intestine.
　▶ **strangulated hernia**：絞扼性（こうやくせい）ヘルニア
　　intestine：腸

☐ MRI検査はC4/5間の椎間板ヘルニアを示しています。
The MRI shows disk herniation between the C4 and C5 vertebrae.
　▶ **disk herniation**：椎間板ヘルニア
　　C4, C5　C=cervical：頸椎の
　　vertebra：椎骨、脊椎骨（複数形：vertebrae）

3 ヘルニア Hernia

処置・手術

- [ ] あなたのヘルニアは実際には非常に小さいものです。こうした症状の場合は私は「経過観察」のアプローチを取りたいと思います。

❋ Your hernia is quite small, actually. This makes me want to take a "wait and see" approach.

- [ ] 穏やかな痛み止めを処方できますよ。これは習慣性のある薬ではありません。痛まないときは服用する必要もありません。

I can prescribe mild painkillers. These are not habit-forming. You don't need to take them when you aren't in pain, either.

- [ ] 残念ながら手術が唯一の解決策だと思います。あなたのヘルニアは大きく、直ちに処置すべきです。

I'm afraid the only solution is surgery. Your hernia is large and should be treated right away.

- [ ] あなたは前立腺の手術をした経験がありますので、腹腔鏡手術には向いていません。私たちはヘルニア整復を開腹術で行う必要があります。

Since you've had prostate surgery in the past, you're not a good candidate for laparoscopy. We need to repair your hernia through open surgery.

▶ laparoscopic：腹腔鏡

- [ ] 直ちに入院していただきたいと思います。私たちは数多くの経験を持っており、開腹手術で成果を挙げています。

I'd like to check you in right away. We have a lot of experience and good results with open surgery.

- [ ] 仕事に早く戻れますから、腹腔鏡手術の方がよろしければ、ヘルニアの手術だけを行う外科医にした方がいいでしょう。

If you prefer the laparoscopic surgery, which would get you back to work much sooner, you are better off with a surgeon that only does hernia surgeries.

- [ ] 看護師が奥様に、ご自宅から必ず持参あるいは購入される物のリストをお渡しします。

The nurse will give you a list of what your wife should bring from home or purchase for you.

Chapter 11 - 整形外科

4 手根管症候群 ... Carpal Tunnel Syndrome

Dr. Katoの元を訪れた患者は長年、手根管症候群を患っています。手術については術後の手を使えない期間を考え、躊躇しています。

Dr. I'm looking at your test results. Let's go over what's going on with your hand. First of all, nerve conduction readings over 5.0 indicate that there's something wrong with your hand. This is your dominant hand, so you've been using it for a variety of tasks … Have you had a carpal tunnel syndrome diagnosis before?

Pt. Yes. Actually, it was more than 30 years ago.

Dr. This is the X-ray of the bones in your hand. The bones are normal, but you drew on the chart that you have tingling in all of your digits except for your little finger, right?

Pt. Yes, that's correct. I don't have any tingling in my pinkie.

Dr. All right. I want you to put the backs of your hands together like this. Does this make your fingers feel worse?

Pt. Maybe.

Dr. Can you put your index finger and thumb together in a circle?

Pt. A circle? Like this?

Dr. That isn't exactly a circle… So, you've been dealing with this issue for a long time. Did you ever consider surgery?

Pt. I've thought about it on and off for many years, but I've been afraid of the recovery time. I do a lot of writing for my job and I can't stop using my hand for six weeks.

Dr. That's very old school. I do endoscopic microsurgery for carpal tunnel here. You would have to avoid bearing a lot of weight for a while, but you'd have normal use of your fingers almost immediately. Here is a handout. It shows the tests we just did and explains the procedure with pictures on the back.

4 手根管症候群　Carpal Tunnel Syndrome

訳

D：検査結果を拝見しています。あなたの手に何が起きているのかを検討しましょう。まず、5.0を超える神経伝導の読み取り値は、あなたの手に何か問題があることを示しています。こちらはあなたの利き手ですから、さまざまな目的に使っていらっしゃいます。今までに手根管症候群になったことはありますか。

P：はい。実は、30年以上前です。

D：これはあなたの手のレントゲン写真です。骨は正常ですが、小指以外の全部の指がうずいていると表に記載しておられますね？

P：はい、その通りです。小指には何のうずきもありません。

D：わかりました。あなたの両方の手の甲を、このようにくっ付けていただけますか。こうすると、それぞれの指の具合が悪くなりますか。

P：たぶん。

D：人差し指と親指で丸が作れますか。

P：丸ですか。こんな具合ですか。

D：それは正確には丸ではありません。それで、あなたは長年、この症状を抱えてきましたね。手術を考えたことはありますか。

P：長年、考えたり考えなかったりでしたが、回復期間のことを懸念していました。仕事で多くの書き物をするので、6週間も手を使うのはやめられません。

D：それは時代遅れです。私はここで手根管の内視鏡顕微鏡手術を行っています。しばらくの間、重いものを持つのを避けなければなりませんが、ほとんどすぐに、指を普通に使えるでしょう。ここに資料があります。私たちが行ったばかりの検査を示しており、裏側に手術の手順を説明してあります。

語句・表現

nerve conduction：神経伝導　＊神経伝導検査（Nerve conduction study）。四肢のしびれや脱力を呈する患者で、末梢神経障害が疑われる場合に行う検査。
readings：読み取り値
dominant hand：利き手
tingling：うずき
digit：（人間の手や足の）指
pinkie：小指
back of one's hand：手の甲
old school：保守的な、古風な
endoscopic：内視鏡の
microsurgery：顕微鏡（下）手術，マイクロサージャリー

整形外科　使える表現

診察・診断

☐ 指に何か痛みやしびれはありますか。
Do you have any pain or numbness in your fingers?

はい。親指と人差し指の具合が非常に悪いです。常にうずきます。中指や薬指が痛むこともあります。
Yeah. It's really bad with my thumb and index finger. They tingle all the time. Sometimes my middle and ring fingers bother me, too.

☐ 小指は大丈夫なのですね。
Your little finger is fine, though, right?

☐ それらは手根管症候群の典型的な症状です。物をギュッとつかむといった場合に力が入らないことはありますか。
Those are classic symptoms. Do you have any weakness, such as having trouble holding onto things?

いつの間にか、物を落とします。
I do find myself dropping things.

☐ 今までに手根管症候群になったことはありますか。
❀ **Have you had a carpal tunnel syndrome diagnosis before?**

☐ 5.0を超える神経伝導の読み取り値は、あなたの手に何か問題があることを示唆しています。
❀ **Nerve conduction readings over 5.0 indicate that there is something wrong with your hand.**

☐ あなたの両方の手の甲を、このようにくっ付けていただけますか。
❀ **I want you to put the backs of your hands together like this.**

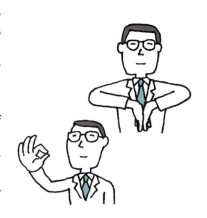

☐ 人差し指と親指で丸が作れますか。
❀ **Can you put your index finger and thumb together in a circle?**

4 手根管症候群 ●●● Carpal Tunnel Syndrome

☐ **Dr.** 手根管症候群の手術を考えたことがありますか。
Have you considered surgery for carpal tunnel syndrome?

Pt. もちろんです。でも、私は手首が使えないで過ごさなければならない時間のことを、とても気にかけています。

Sure. I'm quite concerned about the time I have to spend not being able to use my wrist, though.

手術の紹介・予約

☐ 私はここで手根管の内視鏡顕微鏡手術を行っています。

❋ I do endoscopic microsurgery for carpal tunnel here.

☐ 今月いっぱいは手術の空きがありませんが、たぶん来月の初旬には入れられるでしょう。

We don't have any spaces available for surgery for the rest of this month, but we could probably get you in early next month.

☐ 手術の前に採血が必要になります。手術の前に、病院にお越しいただかなくてよい方をお望みなら、採血を今やることも可能です。

We need to draw blood before the surgery. We can do that now, if you'd prefer not to have to come back before the surgery.

▶ draw blood：採血する

☐ リドカインパッチがありますので、麻酔が投与された時も、針の痛みを感じません。保険が適用されませんので、100円かかります。

We offer a Lidoderm patch so that you don't feel the needle when the anesthesia is administered. It isn't covered by insurance, so that will cost 100 yen.

☐ リドカインパッチは皮膚の表面を麻痺させるだけです。針が刺される間は、たいてい疼痛があります。

The Lidocaine patch only numbs the surface. There is usually continued pain while the needle penetrates the skin.

▶ Lidoderm patch：リドカインパッチ（皮膚表面麻酔剤）
continued pain：疼痛

Chapter 12 - 心臓血管外科

1 虚血性心疾患 ●●● Ischemic Heart Disease

心臓血管外科のDr. Moriを訪れた患者は、肩の痛みで通院していた医院でDr. Moriを紹介されたということです。最近胸の圧迫感も感じるようになっています。

Dr. You say it began with chronic shoulder pain, but then you started feeling chest pressure?

Pt. Yes, I went to see another doctor for the shoulder pain. She tried to treat it, but it didn't go away. Then, I started having the chest issue and she recommended I come talk to you.

Dr. This pressure is on the left side?

Pt. Yes.

Dr. I'd like to do a quick physical. (pause) I'm concerned that we might be dealing with some sort of blockage. I'd like to run tests. First, we should get an ECG.

Pt. Is that different than an EKG?

Dr. No, it's the same test. For some reason, they often use the old German acronym in North America.

Pt. Oh.

Dr. Have you had any other symptoms? Some people experience fatigue.

Pt. Actually, I've been kind of tired lately …

Dr. Since you say this has been going on for a while, I'd like to do this testing right away. Did you walk to the hospital today?

Pt. No, I came by taxi.

Dr. Did you come up here by stairs or on the elevator?

Pt. I took the elevator. Why?

Dr. Sometimes exercise before the test can give us false results. I don't think that's the case here, so we should be able to get an accurate reading.

1 虚血性心疾患　Ischemic Heart Disease

訳

D：慢性的な肩の痛みが始まり、その後胸部の圧迫感を感じ始めたとのことですね。

P：はい、私は肩の痛みで別の医師に診てもらいました。医師は治療を試みましたが、痛みは治まりませんでした。その後、胸の圧迫感が始まりまして、先生に相談しに行くよう勧められました。

D：この圧迫感は左側ですね。

P：はい。

D：簡単に診察してみましょう。(中断) 何らかの閉塞があるのではと懸念しています。検査をしたいと思います。まず、ECG（心電図）をとる必要があります。

P：それはEKGとは違いますか。

D：いいえ、同じ検査です。どういう訳か、北米では昔のドイツ語の頭文字をよく使用します。

P：ああ。

D：他に別の症状はありましたか。疲労感を経験する人がいますが。

P：実は、最近多少疲労感があります。

D：この症状がしばらくの間続いているとのことなので、この検査を直ちに行いたいと思います。今日、病院には歩いて来られましたか。

P：いいえ、タクシーで来ました。

D：ここへは階段で来られましたか、それともエレベータでしたか。

P：エレベーターを使いました。なぜですか。

D：検査前の運動が、時々間違った結果をもたらすことがあります。ここでは、影響ないと思いますので、正確な測定値を得ることができるはずです。

語句・表現

do a quick physical (examination)：簡単に身体診察をする
ECG (elektrokardiogramm)：心電図
acronym：頭文字
accurate reading：正確な測定値

Chapter 12 心臓血管外科

心臓血管外科　使える表現

症状をたずねる

☐ 慢性的な肩の痛みが始まり、その後胸部の圧迫感を感じ始めたとのことですね。
❋ You say it began with chronic shoulder pain, but then you started feeling chest pressure?

☐ 他に別の症状はありましたか。疲労感を経験する人がいますが。
❋ Have you had any other symptoms? Some people experience fatigue.

☐ 病歴と日常の習慣を調べたいと思います。定期的に運動はなさっていますか。
I'd like to go over your medical history and your daily habits. Do you get regular exercise?

☐ 食習慣を教えてください。日常の飲食物には脂肪分が多いですか。
Tell me about your eating habits. Is there a lot of fat in your diet?

☐ 過去にコレステロールが高いと診断されたことはありますか。
Have you been diagnosed with high cholesterol in the past?

☐ カルテによると、しばらくの間高血圧症を患っていて、利尿剤を服用していますね。
According to your chart, you've been dealing with high blood pressure for a while and taking diuretics.

診断

☐ これは我々が「無症候性虚血」と呼んでいるものです。心臓の血流に問題があるのですが、患者には明白な自覚症状がありません。
This is what we call "silent ischemia." There are blood flow issues in the heart, but the patient doesn't experience overt symptoms.
　▶ silent ischemia：無症候性虚血　　overt symptoms：明白な症状

☐ あなたは心筋虚血だと思います。それは血流に関連した心臓疾患です。
I believe you have myocardial ischemia, a heart condition related to blood flow.
　▶ myocardial ischemia：心筋虚血　　heart condition：心臓疾患

1 虚血性心疾患 ●●● Ischemic Heart Disease

処置・処方

☐ 増強型体外式カウンタパルセーションを試したいと思います。切開などの手術は伴いませんが、心臓への血流を改善する効果が期待できます。

We'd like to try enhanced external counterpulsation. It's non-invasive, but can be effective in improving blood flow to the heart.

▶ enhanced external counterpulsation (EECP)：増強型体外式カウンタパルセーション　　non-invasive：非侵襲的　＊皮膚の切開などの手術を伴わないこと。

☐ ステントを入れたいと思います。この治療は最小限の手術によるカテーテル法で行うことが可能です。

I'd like to put in a stent. This procedure can be done with catheterization, which is minimally invasive.

▶ put in a stent：ステントを留置する　　catheterization：カテーテル法
invasive：侵襲的な　＊メスなどで体を傷つけて行う療法。

☐ 検査結果を再検討しましたが、バイパス手術の予定を入れたいと思います。

After reviewing your test results, I'd like to schedule you for bypass surgery.

☐ 最初にやっていただきたいのは、コレステロール降下薬の服用です。この薬は、動脈内に蓄積している原因物質を減らします。

The first thing I'd like to do is put you on cholesterol-lowering medication. This will decrease the primary material that deposits in the arteries.

▶ cholesterol-lowering medication：コレステロール降下薬（高脂血症薬）

☐ β（ベータ）遮断薬を始めたいと思います。この薬は心筋の緩和、心拍数の低下や、血圧の低下を助けます。

I'd like to start you on beta blockers. These will help relax your heart muscle, slow your heart rate and decrease blood pressure.

▶ beta blocker：β（ベータ）遮断薬　　heart muscle：心筋

☐ 利尿剤と共にACE阻害薬を服用していただき、1ヶ月後に再診してください。

I'd like you to try taking the ACE inhibitor along with your diuretics and come back and see me in a month.

▶ ACE (angiotensin-converting enzyme) inhibitor：アンジオテンシン変換酵素抑制剤

Chapter 13 脳神経外科

1 てんかん ••• Epilepsy

脳神経外科の Dr. Nomura は娘がてんかんの発作を起こしたという母親に様子を聞いています。発作は今回が初めてではないようです。

Dr. You say your daughter was having seizures. Would you describe it for me?

P.M. (Patient's mother): My daughter suddenly stopped moving and lost consciousness. And she got a vacant look in her eyes and her eyelids started to flutter.

Dr. Has your daughter had seizures before?

P.M. It happened more than once the other day. The doctor in the emergency room referred us to you.

Dr. Has she had any high fevers recently?

P.M. Yes. We were having trouble keeping her fever down this past week. She had some sort of flu. It scared me when she had the seizure, so I brought her in.

Dr. Did she have any long seizures?

P.M. Not really. I think it was only two times and each was quite short.

Dr. Sometimes high fevers can cause seizures. This usually is not a form of epilepsy. Let's keep an eye on her. According to the nurse, she just has a slight fever now. Hopefully, the virus is on its way out and it will take all of these nasty symptoms with it.

P.M. I hope you're right.

Dr. I'd like you to give her acetaminophen to see if we can keep the fever down. I'll give you a prescription. Give her the recommended daily dose for the next two days. If she isn't a lot better or if she has repeated seizures, please come back to the hospital.

語句・表現

seizure：発作

acetaminophen：アセトアミノフェン（鎮痛剤）

1 てんかん ●●● Epilepsy

訳

D：お嬢さんがけいれん（てんかん）発作を起こされたとのことですが。詳しく説明していただけますか。

PM（患者の母）：突然、動きが止まって意識を失いました。それから、目はうつろになり、まぶたが小きざみに震え始めました。

D：お嬢さんは以前、発作を起こしたことがありますか。

PM：つい先日も複数回起こりました。救急治療室の先生が、先生を紹介してくださいました。

D：お嬢さんは最近、高熱を出したことがありますか。

PM：はい、あります。先週、私たちは娘の熱を下げるのに苦労しました。何らかの風邪だったのです。娘が発作を起こしたとき怖かったので、ここに連れて来ました。

D：お嬢さんには長い発作がありましたか。

PM：別に。発作は2回だけで、とても短かったと思います。

D：高熱が発作を起こすことがあります。この場合、大抵はてんかん型のものではありません。様子を見ましょう。看護師によると、お嬢さんは今、少し熱があるとのことです。できれば、ウイルスが消滅し、ウイルスとともにこうした厄介な症状を全部取り去ってくれるといいのですが。

PM：先生のおっしゃる通りであってほしいです。

D：熱を下げておけるかどうか様子を見るために、アセトアミノフェンを飲ませてください。処方箋を出します。これから2日間、指定する1日の服用量を飲ませてください。もしあまり回復しない、あるいは発作を繰り返すようなら、再診してください。

表現のポイント

epilepsy（てんかん）

「てんかんを起こす」、「てんかん持ちである」は、have epilepsy、have an epileptic seizure。seizure は「発作」、「発作を起こす」という意味の単語で、「てんかん発作」は epileptic seizure、heart seizure は「心臓発作」です。この会話で医師は、まず発作がてんかんによるものか、あるいは別の要因によるものかを診断しています。

脳神経外科　使える表現

症状をたずねる

- [ ] **Dr.** 赤ちゃんが発作を起こしているとのことですが。詳しく説明していただけますか。
  It says your baby is having seizures. Can you describe them for me?
  Pt. 腕と足が四方八方にけいれんするのです。
  His arms and legs jerk all around.

- [ ] お嬢さんは以前、発作を起こしたことがありますか。
  ❇ Has your daughter had seizures before?

- [ ] **Dr.** 発作はどのくらい続きますか。
  How long does it last?
  Pt. 20秒くらいで意識を取り戻して、また、発作の前の動作を続けます。
  She comes to in about 20 seconds and continues doing whatever she was doing before the attack.

- [ ] 彼女は最近高熱を出したことがありますか。
  ❇ Has she had any high fevers recently?

- [ ] 抗けいれん薬の効き目はどんな具合か教えてください。
  Tell me, how have you been doing on the anti-seizure medicine?

診断・処置

- [ ] 高熱が発作を起こすことがあります。この場合、大抵はてんかん型のものではありません。
  ❇ Sometimes high fevers can cause seizures. This usually is not a form of epilepsy.

- [ ] **Pt.** 私の発作の原因は何なのかおわかりでしょうか。
  Have you figured out why I had the seizure to begin with?
  Dr. いいえ、これ以上の情報はありません。私たちはこれまでのところ、あなたの脳内に、この発作の原因となる特定の病変を検知していません。
  No, we don't have any more information. We haven't found any specific lesion in your brain that may be causing this.
  ▶ lesion：病変、傷害

1 てんかん ●●● Epilepsy

- [ ] はっきりした原因が見つからないことはよくあることです。実際には、てんかんのうちの約70%がそうなのです。

  Not finding the exact cause is not that unusual. Actually this occurs in about 70% of epilepsy.

- [ ] ただ、大抵の場合、発作を起こす人は、投薬によって、二度と問題が起こりません。

  Most of the time, though, people have a seizure, take the medication, and they never have the problem again.

- [ ] 熱を下げておけるかどうか様子を見るために、アセトアミノフェンを飲ませてください。

  ❋ I'd like you to give her acetaminophen to see if we can keep the fever down.

- [ ] 胃の不調は、抗けいれん薬でよく起きる副作用です。低用量の薬で始めたので副作用が避けられればよいと思っていたのです。

  Stomach trouble is a common side effect of the anti-seizure medicine. I was hoping that we'd started at a low enough dose to avoid side effects.

子供のけいれん

- [ ] あなたの赤ちゃんの場合、これは単に神経過敏による可能性が高いです。

  In your baby's case, it's more than likely that this is just jitteriness.
  ▶ jitteriness：いら立ち、神経過敏

- [ ] そのようなときは腕や足の位置を変えてみると、いら立ちが和らいだり、場合によっては一気に収まったりするかもしれません。

  If you try changing the position of the baby's arms and legs when he's like that, it may reduce or even stop the jitteriness altogether.

- [ ] 手足の位置を変えるようにし、何が彼をいら立たせているのか、その原因を突き止めるよう試みてください。

  Try altering the position of his limbs and try to get to the bottom of whatever is bothering him.

- [ ] 赤ちゃんの動きを、間代発作と間違える人がよくいます。

  People often mistake the movements of babies for clonic seizures.
  ▶ clonic seizure：間代発作　＊てんかんの全般発作の一つ。全身または一部の筋肉が律動的に攣縮を繰り返す。

Chapter 13 - 脳神経外科

2 脳卒中 ●●● Stroke

脳神経外科のDr. Nomuraは自宅で倒れて救急搬送された患者の奥さんから話を聞いています。

Dr. How long ago did your husband start showing signs of a medical emergency?

P.W. (Patient's wife): We had just finished a late lunch, so I think it was around 2pm.

Dr. So that was about 90 minutes ago. Good. Can you tell me exactly what happened, Mrs. Grossman?

P.W. We were talking about going for a walk after lunch, our typical routine on a Sunday, and he slumped down, groaned and didn't seem to be able to move his right side. I sat him up in the chair and called for an ambulance immediately.

Dr. You did the right thing. There's a window of time after a stroke of about three hours where we can perform the sort of intervention that we want to do with Mr. Grossman successfully. I want to double check something before we administer the drug I have in mind. Is your husband on any heart medication?

P.W. No. His heart is strong, as far as I know.

Dr. Any other medication or allergies?

P.W. He gets hay fever in the spring, but he's not on anything now.

Dr. It doesn't sound like he has anything else going on that will interfere with this. We are going to give him a drug called t-PA. I'll have the nurse start an IV right away.

語句・表現

slump down：崩れるように倒れる
intervention：医療介入
administer the drug：薬を投与する
hay fever：花粉症
t-PA (tissue-plasminogen activator)：組織プラスミノゲン活性化因子（血栓溶解薬）
start an IV：点滴を開始する

訳

D：ご主人の救急を要する事態の兆候はどのくらい前から始まりましたか。

PW（患者の妻）：私たちが遅めのランチを終えてすぐでしたから、午後2時頃だと思います。

D：では90分くらい前ですね。よかった。グロスマンさん、何が起きたのか正確に教えていただけますか。

PW：私たちが日曜日はいつも日課の、昼食後の散歩について話していたら、主人が崩れるように倒れ、うなり、右側が動かせないように見えました。私は主人を起こして椅子に座らせすぐに救急車を呼びました。

D：適切な処置でしたね。脳卒中発症後にはある程度介入できる約3時間の時間枠がありますので、グロスマンさんにはうまく処置したいと思っています。私が考えている薬を投与する前に、いくつか再確認したいと思います。ご主人は何かの薬物治療を受けていますか。

PW：いいえ、私が知る限り、心臓は強いです。

D：他に何か薬を服用していたり、アレルギーがあったりしますか。

PW：主人は春、花粉症がありますが、今は何もありません。

D：この薬を投与しても差し支えないようですね。t-PAという薬を処方します。すぐに看護師に点滴を開始してもらいましょう。

雑学
脳卒中の症状を確かめる3つの検査

1. **Ask the person to smile.**　笑ってもらう
（顔面の麻痺）　片方の顔面が反対側に比べて動きが悪い。
2. **Ask the person to raise both arms.**　両腕を挙げてもらう
（腕の異常）　一方の手が挙がらない。挙げても下方に変位する。
3. **Ask the person to speak a simple sentence.**　短文を話してもらう
（言語の異常）　不明瞭な発語を使う。またはまったくしゃべれない。

脳神経外科　使える表現

症状をたずねる

☐ **Dr.** 何が起きたのか教えていただけますか。
❋ Can you tell me what happened?

P.S. 父が脳卒中を起こしているようなのです。話すのが困難で、体の半分がまひしているように見えます。

I think my father is having a stroke. He's having trouble talking and one side of his body seems paralyzed.
▶ paralyzed：麻痺した

☐ ご主人の救急を要する事態の兆候はどのくらい前から始まりましたか。
❋ How long ago did your husband start showing signs of a medical emergency?

☐ ご主人は何か心臓の薬物治療を受けていますか。
❋ Is your husband on any heart medication?

診察

☐ 非常に簡単な検査をいくつか行います。笑ってもらえますか。
I want to do some very simple tests. Could I ask you smile?

☐ 両腕を挙げていただけますか。
Could you raise both of your arms up in the air?

☐ 短い文を一つか二つ話していただけますか。ご自分のことを少し話してください。
I need you to speak a simple sentence or two. Tell me a little bit about yourself.

☐ 卒中を起こしていると思いますので、待っていらっしゃる方々よりも先に（処置室へ）お連れします。
I believe you've had a stroke, so I'm going to take you in front of the rest of these people.
▶ have a stroke：卒中を起こす

手術後の家族への説明

☐ 奥様は今手術が終わったところです。診察室に戻って話しましょう。

Your wife is out of surgery now. Let's go back to my office to talk.

☐ ゴールドさんは脳に動脈瘤がありました。緊急手術を行い、塊を取り除きました。しかしながら、今は昏睡状態です。

Mr. Gold had a brain aneurism. We did emergency surgery and removed the clot. However, he's in a coma now.
▶ aneurism：動脈瘤 　 clot：塊 　 in a coma：昏睡状態で

☐ 彼女は極めて深刻な脳の損傷を被ってこられましたが、私たちは回復にとても期待を持っています。

She's been through extremely serious brain trauma, but we are very hopeful that she will recover.
▶ brain trauma：脳損傷

☐ 理学療法を続ければ、いずれ身体のそちら半分の側も動かせるようになると思います。

I believe that if he keeps up with the physical therapy he'll eventually be able to move that side of his body, as well.
▶ physical therapy：理学療法

☐ 4週間以上昏睡状態にある人はめったにありませんが、4週間昏睡状態だった私の患者さんは、今とても元気です。

People are rarely in comas for more than four weeks, but my patient that was in a coma for that long is doing quite well now.

表現のポイント

患者が脳卒中を説明する症状
- ★ I have a terrible headache for apparently no reason.
  明らかに原因不明の激しい頭痛があります。
- ★ My vision is blurred. 　視界がぼやけます。
  ▶ blurred：不鮮明な、ぼやけた
- ★ It's hard to speak clearly. 　はっきり話すのが困難です。
- ★ I'm numb on this side of my body. (pointing)
  （場所を指し示しながら）体のこちらの側がしびれています。

Chapter 13 - 脳神経外科

3　アルツハイマー病 ●●● Alzheimer's Disease

脳神経外科の Dr. Nomura は物忘れで受診した患者と付き添いの娘さんから話を聞いています。物忘れは、1年ほど前からのようです。

Dr. Good morning, I'm Doctor Nomura.

P.D. (Patient's daughter): It's nice to meet you. You come highly recommended. This is my mother, Ellen Harris. I'm Grace. We moved here a few months ago. Her memory's been a bit <u>foggy</u> for about a year now.

Pt. My memory is just fine.

Dr. Ms. Harris, I'm going to say three words and I want you to listen and then repeat them back to me when I say "What were the words?." Okay?

Pt. Sure.

Dr. Dish … bicycle … love. Okay, what were the words?

Pt. Love … uh … bicycle … (pause)

Dr. There was one more word …

Pt. I can't remember.

Dr. No problem.

Dr. Did your mother have a <u>neurological work-up</u> in the U.S.?

P.D. Not really. It took us a while to catch on and then we were gearing up to move here.

Dr. There are some more sophisticated <u>neurological tests</u> that we can do. I also want to look at some other possible issues. Sometimes nutrition, <u>dehydration</u> and <u>thyroid</u> issues play a part when there are memory issues. I have access to information about them in English and I can get English versions of questions we need to ask. Would you like to make an appointment for that?

P.D. Yes, we'd like that.

3 アルツハイマー病 ●●● Alzheimer's Disease

訳

D： おはようございます。野村です。

PD：（患者の娘）：お会い出来て光栄です。先生を紹介されて伺いました。こちらは母のエレン・ハリス。私はグレースです。私たちは数ヶ月前にここに越してきました。1年ほど前から母の記憶力があまりはっきりしていません。

P： 私の記憶力はしっかりしているよ。

D： ハリスさん、これから3つの単語を言いますのでそれを聞いて、私が「単語は何でしたか」とたずねたら、繰り返して言ってもらえますか。いいですか。

P： はい。

D： Dish, bicycle, love. では、単語は何でしたか。

P： Love …、えーと bicycle…。（中断）

D： もう1つ単語がありましたね。

P： 覚えていません。

D： 大丈夫ですよ。

D： お母様は米国で神経学的な検査を受けられましたか。

PD： 特には受けていません。症状を理解するまでにしばらく時間がかかり、その上日本に越してくる準備がありましたので。

D： より高度な神経学的検査をいくつか提供できます。私は他に考えられる問題点も見てみたいと思います。記憶力の低下には、栄養不足や脱水症状や甲状腺の疾患といった問題が関わっている場合があります。そうした情報を英語で得ていますので、質問事項の英語版も入手できます。検査の予約をなさいませんか。

PD： はい、よろしくお願いします。

語句・表現

foggy：はっきりしない
neurological work-up / test：神経学的検査
dehydration：脱水
thyroid：甲状腺

脳神経外科　使える表現

診察

☐ これから3つの単語を言いますのでそれを聞いて、私が「単語は何でしたか」とたずねたら、繰り返して言ってもらえますか。

❋ I'm going to say three words and I want you to listen and then repeat them back to me when I say "What were the words?."

☐ よく悲しい気持ちになりますよね。これは珍しいことではありません。

I understand you often feel sad. This is not unusual.

☐ 記憶力に何らかの問題があるのですね。そのことでいらいらされるのはわかります。

I understand you've had some memory trouble. I know that can be frustrating.

診断

☐ あなたのお母様は初期のアルツハイマー型認知症です。

Your mother has early stage Alzheimer's dementia.
▶ dementia：認知症

☐ この症状が認知症だとは断定しかねます。物忘れはビタミンの欠乏や甲状腺の疾患が原因の可能性があります。

I'm not positive that this is dementia. Memory loss can be caused by vitamin deficiencies or thyroid disease.

処置・処方・助言

☐ 記憶力の低下には、栄養不足や脱水症状や甲状腺の疾患といった問題が関わっている場合があります。

❋ Sometimes nutrition, dehydration and thyroid issues play a part when there are memory issues.

☐ 今日診察に来られたとき、お母様は脱水状態でした。十分に水分をとって物忘れが改善した患者さんがいらっしゃいます。

Your mother was dehydrated when she came in today. I've had patients whose memories were better when they were properly hydrated.

> dehydrated：脱水状態の

☐ 遅い時間帯にカフェイン入りの飲み物も飲まないようにするとよいかもしれません。カフェイン入りの飲み物で、夜に眠れなくなることがあります。

You may want to avoid drinking anything with caffeine in it later in the day. Drinks with caffeine often make it hard to fall asleep at night.

☐ ご家族があなたをもっといろいろな活動に誘ってくださるでしょう。もっと運動をしていただきたいと思います。

Maybe your family can get you involved in more activities. I want you to get more exercise.

☐ 奥様の場合、栄養面に問題があると思います。特にフルーツや野菜といった自然食品や健康食品をもっと食べる必要があります。

In your wife's case, I think we're seeing nutritional issues at play. She needs to be eating more, especially whole, healthy foods, such as fruits and vegetables.

> at play：作動中の　　whole food：自然食品

☐ より高度な神経学的検査をいくつか提供できます。

✱ There are some more sophisticated neurological tests that we can do.

☐ 神経学的検査は特にアルツハイマー病の初期段階に有益です。今後記憶障害を記録していくのに利用できる基準にもなります。

Neurological testing is especially valuable in the early stages of Alzheimer's. It can give us a baseline we can use to chart future memory loss, as well.

☐ アリセプトという薬を処方しましょう。アリセプトはアルツハイマー病が原因の軽度から中程度の認知症を治療するのに用いられます。

Let me prescribe a medicine called Aricept. Aricept is used to treat mild to moderate dementia caused by Alzheimer's disease.

Chapter 14 - 乳腺外科

1　乳腺腫瘍　●●● Breast Growths

乳腺外科の Dr. Ono は胸にしこりのあるのを見つけ、心配して来院した患者を診察しています。

Dr. Good morning, Ms. Wilson. What brings you to the hosptial today?

Pt. I was doing a self-exam and I discovered a lump.

Dr. I see. I'll have the nurse bring you a gown. I'd like to take a look and palpate it. (pause) Could you show me exactly where this is?

Pt. Here.

Dr. Ah. According to the chart, your last mammogram was about nine months ago … Is that right?

Pt. Yes.

Dr. I'd like to do an ultrasound. Please come with me to the next room.

Pt. Okay.

(Pause)

Dr. All right, please lie back down and hold still for me. This looks like a fluid-filled cyst, but I'd like to aspirate with a needle to be sure. Actually, if I'm right, we may be able to remove the fluid with the needle.

Pt. Oh, that's good.

Dr. The nurse will be back in a minute with what we need.

(Pause)

Dr. It does seem to be fluid. Chances are good that this will completely disappear, but I'd like you to come back in a few weeks to take a look at it again.

1 乳腺腫瘍　●●● Breast Growths

訳

D：ウィルソンさん、おはようございます。今日はこの病院にどういう経緯で来られましたか。

P：自己検診（セルフチェック）をしていたら、しこりを見つけました。

D：なるほど。看護師にガウンを持ってこさせます。拝見して触診したいと思います。（中断）しこりが正確にどこにあるか教えていただけますか。

P：ここです。

D：ああ。カルテによるとあなたが最後に乳房X線撮影をなさったのは9ヶ月前で、正しいですか。

P：はい。

D：超音波検査を行いたいと思います。私と一緒に隣の部屋に来てください。

P：はい。

（中断）

D：さて、あおむけに横になってじっとしていていただけますか。これは液状の嚢腫（のうしゅ）のようですが、念のために針を刺して吸引したいと思います。実際のところ、私の診断が正しければ、針で液体を取り除くことができるでしょう。

P：まあ、それはいいですね。

D：看護師が必要なものを持ってすぐに戻ってきます。

（中断）

D：これはやはり液体のようです。これが完全に消える見込みは大きいですが、もう一度診察したいので、数週間後に再受診してください。

語句・表現

self-exam：自己検診（セルフチェック）
lump：腫れ物、しこり
palpate：〜を触診する
mammogram：マンモグラフィー、乳房X線撮影

ultrasound：超音波
fluid-filled：液体で満たされた
cyst：嚢腫（のうしゅ）
aspirate：吸引する

Chapter 14 乳腺外科

●●● 乳腺外科　使える表現

症状をたずねる

☐ **Dr.** 診断申込書で乳がんの病歴に言及されていますね。

 I see that you mention a history of breast cancer on the form.

Pt. 腫瘍摘出手術を5年前に受けました。母が乳がんで亡くなりましたので、とても注意深く自分で観察してきました。

 I had a lumpectomy five years ago. My mother died of breast cancer, so I've been monitoring myself quite carefully.

 ▶ lumpectomy：腫瘍摘出手術

☐ **Dr.** 自己検診は非常に重要でよいことです。あなたは手術後、どんな治療をなさいましたか。

 Self-monitoring is very important; that's good. What sort of therapies did you have after the surgery?

Pt. 毎日の放射線治療を1ヶ月受けました。

 I had a month of daily radiation.

 ▶ radiation：放射線治療

☐ それ（しこり）が正確にどこにあるか教えていただけますか。

❇ Could you show me exactly where this is?

☐ がんを早期に発見されたようですね。

 It sounds like they caught cancer early.

 ▶ catch cancer early：がんを早期に発見する

検査・診断

☐ これは液状の嚢腫（のうしゅ）のようですが、念のために針を刺して吸引したいと思います。

❇ This looks like a fluid-filled cyst, but I'd like to aspirate with a needle to be sure.

☐ 私の診断が正しければ、針で液体を取り除くことができるでしょう。

❇ If I'm right, we may be able to remove the fluid with the needle.

1 乳腺腫瘍 ●●● Breast Growths

☐ 乳房X線撮影とその後の検査はすべて正常だったようです。

It looks like your mammogram and the subsequent tests were all clean.

☐ 検査結果は腫瘍が悪性であることを示していますが、これはまだステージ1、あるいはステージ0と同等です。

The tests indicate that the tumor is malignant, but this is still stage 1 or even stage 0.
  ▶ malignant：悪性の

☐ 検査結果によるとステージ3であり、悪性腫瘍がリンパ節に転移しています。

The tests have shown that this is stage 3 and that the malignancy has traveled to the lymph nodes.
  ▶ malignancy：悪性腫瘍　　lymph node：リンパ節

治療・助言

☐ あなたの場合、がんの部分を取り除き、乳房は温存する腫瘍摘出手術が可能です。

In your case, we can perform a lumpectomy, where we remove the cancerous areas and leave the breast intact.
  ▶ cancerous：がん（性）の　　intact：損なわれていない、無傷の

☐ 腫瘍マーカーの検査結果は、ER（エストロゲン受容体）陽性でした。この結果は、あなたの場合、ホルモン治療が効果的である可能性が高いことを示しています。

We tested you for tumor markers and you tested ER-positive. This indicates that hormonal therapy is likely to be effective in your case.
  ▶ tumor marker：腫瘍マーカー
　　ER(estrogen-receptor)-positive：エストロゲン受容体陽性（乳がん）

☐ がんの再発を確実に阻止するため、一連の放射線治療と、その後のホルモン治療での経過観察をお願いします。

We'd like to order a round of radiation and then follow-up with hormone therapy to make sure that the cancer does not return.

Chapter 15 - 小児科

1　ぜんそく・インフルエンザ　●●● Asthma/Flu

小児科の Dr. Rikiishi の診察室には、小さい子どもを伴った母親が来ています。ゼーゼーと苦しそうに咳をする幼い息子のことが心配です。　CD2-31

Dr. So, your son is six, is that right, Mrs. Perkins?

P.M. (Patient's mother): Yes. He turned six last month.

Dr. Has he ever been diagnosed with asthma before?

P.M. Asthma? You think he has asthma?

Dr. I need to do a full exam, but he does seem to be wheezing. We usually don't see this kind of extreme breathing issue when it's just the flu. Have you noticed any changes in his mood?

P.M. Uh … maybe he's been a little moody.

Dr. So, he seems upset ... irritable?

P.M. Yes, I'd say he's been kind of grouchy the last few weeks, especially right when he wakes up. He's also been sleeping a lot.

Dr. He seems a little short of breath right now. Have you noticed this before?

P.M. That's also been going on for a couple of weeks. He seems to have a little trouble catching his breath sometimes.

Dr. These are all possible signs of asthma. Since he's six, we can do regular lung function tests. I'd like you both to go with our nurse and she'll conduct some spirometry and other tests and we can discuss the results and treatment options after that.

語句・表現

asthma：ぜんそく
wheeze：苦しそうに息をする
moody：ふさぎ込んだ、不機嫌な
upset：腹を立てて、ブスッとして

irritable：いらいらして
I'd say (I would say) ～：～だろうと思います
＊発言を和らげる表現。say の他に think や

1 ぜんそく・インフルエンザ　Asthma / Flu

訳

D：それで、パーキンスさん、息子さんは6歳でよろしいですね。

PM（患者の母）：はい。先月6歳になりました。

D：今まで、息子さんはぜんそくと診断されたことはありますか。

PM：ぜんそくですか。先生は息子がぜんそくだと思われますか。

D：あらゆる検査を行う必要があります。しかし息子さんはゼーゼーと苦しそうに息をしているようです。通常こうした極端な呼吸の症状は、単なるインフルエンザの場合には見られません。心的な状態に何か変わったことに気づかれましたか。

PM：あのー、少し不機嫌なようでした。

D：それで息子さんは機嫌が悪く、いらいらしているように見えたんですね。

PM：ええ、息子はここ数週間、特に朝起きてすぐの時に機嫌が悪かったと思います。それによく眠っています。

D：息子さんは現在、少々呼吸困難があるようです。今までにこうした症状に気づいたことはありますか。

PM：その症状も2、3週間続いています。ときどき息を整えるのに少し苦労をしているようです。

D：それらはすべて、ぜんそくに起こり得る兆候です。息子さんは6歳ですから、標準の肺機能検査を行うことができます。お二人で看護師のところへ行ってください。看護師が肺活量測定やその他の検査をしますので、その後で、検査結果や治療の選択肢を相談します。

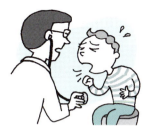

---

　　guessも使われる。
grouchy：機嫌の悪い
short of breath：息を切らして、息切れして
catch one's breath：息を整える

possible sign：起こり得る兆候
spirometry：肺活量測定

Chapter 15 小児科

● ● ● 小児科　使える表現

診察

- 息子さんはぜんそくと診断されたことがありますか。

✤ Has he ever been diagnosed with asthma before?

- 彼は現在、少々呼吸困難があるようです。今までにこうした症状に気づいたことはありますか。

✤ He seems a little short of breath right now. Have you noticed this before?

- **Dr.** こんにちは。今日はどうしたの。

    Hi there. What seems to be the matter today?

    Pt. ちょっと風邪をひいて熱があります。2日間続いています。

    I have some kind of cold and a fever. It's been going on for two days.

- 診てみましょう。「あー」と言って。喉が少し赤いようだね。鼻が詰まっているようだ。頭は痛いかな。

    Let's have a look. Say "ah" ... Your throat is a little red. You sound a bit stuffed up. Does your head hurt?

- 胃の具合はどうかな。食欲不振や下痢はあるかな。

    How about your stomach? Any trouble eating or diarrhea?

診断・処置

- 流行のインフルエンザのようですね。インフルエンザの予防接種は受けましたか。

    This looks like the flu that's been going around. Did he have a flu shot?

- **Dr.** 息子さんが予防接種を受けないのには何か特別な理由がありますか。

    Any particular reason why your son hasn't had a flu shot?

    Pt. ええ、アレルギーがあるので、故郷の先生は受けないようにするべきだと判断されました。

    Yeah, he has allergies, so the doctors back home decided he shouldn't have one.

1 ぜんそく・インフルエンザ ●●● Asthma/Flu

☐ お嬢さんのインフルエンザの症状に対して私たちができることはあまりありませんが、1つ薬を処方します。十分に休ませて、水分をたっぷりとるよう勧めてください。

There isn't much we can do for your daughter's flu symptoms, but I'm prescribing one medication. See that she gets plenty of rest and encourage her to take in lots of fluids.

☐ 息子さんの熱のことが少々心配です。家にお帰りする前に、熱を下げる必要があります。脱水症状もあると思います。

I'm a bit worried about your son's fever. It needs to come down before we can release him. I also think he's dehydrated.
▶ dehydrated：脱水状態の

☐ 息子さんに点滴を行い、看護師には額に冷湿布をあててもらいます。

I'd like to give him some IV fluids and have the nurse apply cool compresses to his forehead.
▶ IV fluid (intravenous fluid)：静脈内輸液、点滴剤　　cool compresses：冷湿布

☐ 点滴が終わる時間までに、熱が正常値に近くならない場合は、たぶん一晩入院された方がよいでしょう。

If we don't see his fever get closer to normal by the time the drip finishes, I probably will recommend admitting him for the night.
▶ drip：点滴

処方・助言

☐ ご両親が薬局で受け取れる薬を処方するけれど、一番よいのは、君が家に帰って2、3日、のんびりすることだね。

I'll prescribe something that your parents can pick up at the pharmacy, but the best thing is for you to go home and take it easy for a few days.

☐ **P.M.** 娘が食べたらよい何かお勧めのものはありますか。

Do you have any recommendations about what my daughter should eat?

Dr. BRAT食をお勧めします。その食事療法は、b-r-a-tと呼ばれます。バナナ (bananas)、米 (rice)、リンゴのすり下ろし (apples sause)、トースト (toast) の略です。

I recommend the BRAT diet. The diet is called b-r-a-t. It stands for bananas, rice apple sauce and toast.

Chapter 16 - 肛門科

1 痔核 ●●● Hemorrhoids

女性にとって肛門科を訪れるのは勇気がいるものです。Dr. Saito は意を決して訪ねてきた患者を丁寧に診察します。

Dr. Hello. So, what brings you here today?

Pt. I've been noticing blood in my stool recently.

Dr. Can you tell if it's bright red?

Pt. I'm not so sure. If I had to guess, I'd say it's kind of bright. I don't see it all the time. It's occasional.

Dr. I'd like to do an exam. Could you put on this gown so that it opens in the back? I'll be back in a second. (pause) All right, I need you to lie down on your left side on the table here. I'm going to do a digital exam first. (pause) Now I'm going to use an anoscope to get a better look. You may feel a little pressure. You can sit up now. You have hemorrhoids.

Pt. Hemorrhoids? What do I need to do?

Dr. At this point, I'd like to recommend that you increase the fiber in your diet and make sure you are drinking plenty of water. I'd also like to suggest sitz baths. This will reduce the swelling. I'm going to prescribe a salve that you can use twice a day for the next two weeks. Are you feeling any pain with this?

Pt. Yes, actually.

Dr. I'll also prescribe acetaminophen to help with that. If you don't feel a lot better in two weeks, please come back and see me.

語句・表現

stool：排泄物
lie (down) on one's left side.：左側を下に横になる
digital exam (examination)：指診
anoscope：肛門鏡、直腸鏡
sitz bath：座浴

1 痔核 ●●● **Hemorrhoids**

訳

D： こんにちは。それで、今日はどうなさいましたか。

P： 最近、排泄物に血が混じるのに気がつきました。

D： 明るい赤色かどうかわかりますか。

P： よくわかりません。どちらかと言えば、やや明るい色だろうと思います。いつもあるわけではないので。見るのは時折です。

D： 検査を行いたいと思います。後ろが開くこのガウンを着用していただけますか。すぐに戻ります。（中断）よろしいですか、ここの台の上で左側を下にして横になってください。最初に指診を行います。（中断）では、もっとよく見るため、これから肛門鏡を使います。少し痛みを感じるかもしれません。起きて結構です。痔核がありますね。

P： 痔核ですか。私はどうすればいいですか。

D： この時点では、食物繊維の多い食事をとることをお勧めしたいと思います。必ず水をたっぷり飲んでください。座浴もお勧めします。これを行うと腫れものが小さくなります。軟膏を処方しますので、これから2週間、1日に2回使用してください。この症状で何か痛みはありますか。

P： はい、実は。

D： その症状の緩和のため、アセトアミノフェンも処方します。2週間であまりよくならなければ、診察にいらしてください。

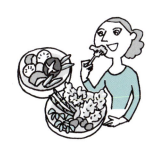

swelling：腫れもの
salve：軟膏
acetaminophen：アセトアミノフェン（炎症を伴わない軽度の痛みのための鎮痛剤）

肛門科　使える表現

症状をたずねる

☐ **Dr.** 症状を説明していただけますか。
　Could you describe the issue for me?
Pt. 排便後に何かがはみ出ているようなのに気がつきました。
I've been noticing after a bowel movement that something is kind of protruding.
　▶ protrude：はみ出る、突き出る

☐ それを押し戻すことはできますか。
Are you able to push it back in?

☐ 明るい赤色かどうかわかりますか。
❇ Can you tell if it's bright red?

☐ **Dr.** この痛みにいつ気づかれましたか。
When did you notice this pain?
Pt. 1週間ほど前に気がつきました。トイレットペーパーに血がついているのにも気がつきました。
I just noticed it about a week ago. I also saw some blood on the toilet paper.

診察

☐ ここの台の上で左側を下に横になってください。最初に指診を行います。
❇ I need you to lie on your left side on the table here. I'm going to do a digital exam first.

☐ もっとよく見るため、これから肛門鏡を使います。少し痛みを感じるかもしれません。
❇ I'm going to use an anoscope to get a better look. You may feel a little pressure.

☐ ビデオ肛門鏡を使って、痔核の状態を実際に記録できます。
Using video anoscopy, we can actually record what's going on with your hemorrhoids.
　▶ anoscopy：肛門鏡検査（法）

1 痔核 ●●● Hemorrhoids

処置

☐ 内痔核にも外痔核にも腫れがあるので、痔核切除をするべきでしょう。

Since we are dealing with both internal and external hemorrhoids, I believe you should have a hemorrhoidectomy.
▶ hemorrhoidectomy：痔核切除

☐ あなたの具体的な症状からすると、手術が最良の選択肢だと思います。

Based on your specific symptoms, I think surgery is your best option.

☐ **Pt.** これらの突出物ががん性の可能性はありますか。

Is there any chance that these protrusions are cancerous?

Dr. 痔核がありますが、悪性腫瘍である可能性はほとんどないと思います。

I think that you have hemorrhoids and that there is little chance of a malignancy.
▶ malignancy：悪性腫瘍

☐ ゴム輪結紮療法を行います。これは全身麻酔をせずに行える比較的簡単な処置です。

I'd like to perform a rubber band ligation. It's a relatively simple procedure that we can perform without general anesthesia.
▶ rubber band ligation：ゴム輪結紮療法　　general anesthesia：全身麻酔

☐ 手術と違って、大部分の日常的な活動にはほとんどすぐに戻ることができます。お願いしたいのは、重いものを持ち上げるのを避けることだけです。

Unlike surgery, you'll be able to return to most of your daily activities pretty much right away. The only thing we'll ask you to avoid is heavy lifting.

助言

☐ 食物繊維の多い食事をとることをお勧めしたいと思います。必ず水をたっぷり飲んでください。

❀ I'd like to recommend that you increase the fiber in your diet and make sure that you are drinking plenty of water.

☐ 座浴もお勧めします。

❀ I'd also like to suggest sitz baths.

Chapter 17 産婦人科

1 子宮筋腫 ●●● Fibroids

先に行った検査結果を聞くため、患者が産婦人科のDr. Tanakaの診察室を訪れます。子宮筋腫の疑いがあり、Dr. Tanakaは治療方針を説明します。

Dr. Based on the exam we just did, I suspect you have fibroids.

Pt. Those aren't cancerous, right?

Dr. It's rare for them to be malignant. In my experience, they're almost always benign. I'd like to schedule some imaging so that we can get a look and decide the course of treatment.

Pt. So, I need an ultrasound?

Dr. Recent research has shown that if we go ahead and do an MRI, we can make better treatment decisions.

Pt. Aren't MRIs expensive?

Dr. They are more costly, but your insurance will cover some of it. I think the cost in Japan is less than what you're used to back in the States. A well-known doctor in my field said that using an MRI instead of an ultrasound was "like listening to a digital CD rather than a record," because "the quality is better in every way."

Pt. Well that certainly is a clear explanation.

Dr. There is a non-surgical technique to, if you will, kill off the tumor called embolization. The MRI lets us evaluate the tumor to see if it's right for that modality.

Pt. Of course, I'd like to avoid surgery, if possible.

Dr. Embolization is non-surgical, but it can be quite painful and may require an overnight stay in the hospital for observation. Anyhow, let's go ahead and do the MRI. If they're smaller than I think they are, we can take a "wait and see" approach.

1 子宮筋腫 ●●● Fibroids

訳

D：今行った検査からすると、子宮筋腫の疑いがありますね。

P：それはがん性ではありませんよね。

D：悪性であることは極めてまれです。私の経験では、ほとんどの場合良性です。いくつかの画像撮影の予定を決めたいと思います。そうすれば、目で見て治療方針を決定できます。

P：それで、私は超音波検査を受ける必要がありますか。

D：最近の研究から、MRI検査を行えば、よりよい治療法が決められることがわかっています。

P：MRIは高額ではありませんか。

D：MRIはより高額ですが、保険でいくらか補填できるでしょう。日本での金額は、米国で支払っていた金額よりも安いと思います。この病気の分野で有名な医師が超音波検査ではなくMRIを使うと、「質があらゆる面で優れている」ので「レコードではなくデジタルCDを聞いているようだ」とおっしゃいました。

P：なるほど、それはわかりやすい説明ですね。

D：もし希望なさるのでしたら、腫瘍を全滅させる塞栓術という、手術を行わない技術があります。MRI検査を行うことで、腫瘍がその治療法に適しているかを判断できます。

P：もちろん、できれば手術は避けたいです。

D：塞栓術は外科的なものではありませんが、大きな痛みを伴い、観察のために一晩の入院が必要となるでしょう。いずれにせよ、MRIを行いましょう。もし大きさが思ったよりも小さければ、経過観察で対応できるでしょう。

語句・表現

cancerous：がんの、がん性の
malignant：悪性の
benign：良性の
ultrasound：超音波検査
MRI (magnetic resonance imaging)：磁気共鳴映像法

non-surgical：手術を行わない
embolization：塞栓術
be right for ～：～に適している
modality：治療法
"wait and see" approach：経過観察（静観しながらのアプローチ）

産婦人科　使える表現

症状をたずねる

□ **Dr.** 生理は規則的ですか。
　Is your menstruation regular?
Pt. 実は、ずっと不順です。
　Actually, it's been irregular.
Dr. 不正出血やおりものはありますか。
　Have you noticed any unusual bleeding or discharge?
　▶ discharge：分泌

□ **Dr.** うまく回復しているようですね。ほてりはありますか。
　It looks like everything is healing nicely. Have you been experiencing any hot flashes?
Pt. はい、ひどい状態です。何度も悩まされていて、時には1時間に4、5回起こります。
　Yes, it's horrible. I'm having them very often, sometimes four or five times an hour.
　▶ hot flash：ホットフラッシュ、ほてり

診断・処置

□ 今行った検査からすると、子宮筋腫の疑いがありますね。
✪ Based on the exam we just did, I suspect you have fibroids.

□ 検査の結果、子宮筋腫との結果が出ました。これは、子宮の筋肉がこぶ状に増殖したものです。よく見られる病気で、女性の4人に1人くらいの割合で起こります。
　The results of the test show that you have fibroids. It's just uterine muscle that's overgrown and formed a mass. It's a common disease and occurs in about 1 in 4 women.

□ 悪性であることは極めてまれです。私の経験では、ほとんどの場合良性です。
✪ It's rare for them to be malignant. In my experience, they're almost always benign.

□ あなたの場合、まだ筋腫が小さいので、経過観察のアプローチをとりたいと思います。
　Your tumor is still small, so I'd like to take a "wait and see" approach.

1 子宮筋腫 ●●● Fibroids

- [ ] 処方したホルモン補充薬が、効くべきレベルに作用していないようです。別の薬を試したいと思います。

  I guess the hormone replacement medicine we prescribed is not working as well as it should. I'd like to try another medication.
  - ▶ hormone replacement：ホルモン補充

- [ ] もし希望なさるのでしたら、腫瘍を全滅させる塞栓術という、手術を行わない技術があります。

  ❂ There is a non-surgical technique to, if you will, kill off the tumor called embolization.

子宮摘出

- [ ] MRIの検査結果を詳細に調べましたが、あなたの子宮筋腫のサイズや性質からして、子宮の完全摘出をお勧めします。

  I've been over your MRI and my recommendation, based on the size and nature of the fibroids, is a complete hysterectomy.
  - ▶ complete hysterectomy：子宮の完全摘出

- [ ] この種の腫瘍は罹患した臓器を取り除かなければ再発する可能性が非常に高いです。

  This type of tumor is very likely to come back unless we remove the affected organs.

- [ ] **Dr.** まだ出産はお考えですか。

  Do you still have reproductive plans?

  Pt. いいえ、私は45歳で十代の息子がいますから、もう子供は考えていません。

  No, I'm 45 and we have a teenage son, so I wasn't planning on having any more children.
  - ▶ reproductive plan：出産計画

- [ ] 再来週に塞栓術の予定を入れたいと思います。

  We'd like to schedule you for an embolization the week after next.

- [ ] 大事をとって、がん専門医に立ち会ってもらいたいと思います。

  We like to have an oncologist on hand just to be on the safe side.
  - ▶ oncologist：がん（腫瘍）専門医　　on the safe side：大事をとって

2 分娩 ... Childbirth

今日、産婦人科の Dr. Tanaka が診察している患者は日本に引っ越してきたばかり。日本で初出産を迎えます。

Dr. Your records indicated you're just entering your second trimester. You had your original prenatal care in New Zealand?

Pt. Yes, that's where were from. We just moved here last month.

Dr. So then you'll be giving birth here? Is this your first child?

Pt. Correct.

Dr. And did the nurse give you the information sheets we have in English?

Pt. Yes, I got them, thank you.

Dr. Let's check your blood pressure first. (pause) Next, I'd like to examine your belly. I'm going to record some measurements.

Pt. I'm worried about the weight gain. I already feel huge.

Dr. I can see that you were underweight when all this began. In women like you, we really encourage weight gain.

Pt. Really? I've heard that Japanese doctors often tell foreign women they're gaining too much weight.

Dr. Every case is different. Gaining a half kilo to a kilogram per month is normal. As I said, because you began your pregnancy on the lean side, you could gain more without being concerned. It can be a strange sensation for small women, but you're providing a home for your baby, this is no time to diet.

Pt. Oh, of course not.

Dr. Let's listen to the baby's heart rate with the heart rate Doppler. … Everything sounds fine to me.

2 分娩 ●●● Childbirth

訳

D：記録によると、ちょうど妊娠中期に入ったところですね。最初の妊婦検診はニュージーランドでなさったのですね。

P：はい、そのニュージーランドから来ました。私たちは先月ここに引っ越してきたばかりです。

D：では、ここで出産なさるということですね。最初のお子さんですか。

P：そうです。

D：それで看護師があなたに当院の英語版情報シートをお渡ししましたか。

P：はい、いただきました。ありがとうございます。

D：まず血圧を測りましょう。（中断）次に、腹部を検査したいと思います。いくつか測定の記録を取ります。

P：私は体重が増えていることを心配しています。すでにすごく体が大きくなっているように感じます。

D：妊娠初期は体重不足だったのですね。あなたのような女性には、私たちはぜひ体重を増やすようお勧めしています。

P：本当ですか。日本人のお医者さんは外国人の女性に、体重が増えすぎているとよくおっしゃるのだと聞いたことがあります。

D：ケースによって異なります。1ヶ月に0.5kgから1kg増えるのは正常です。申し上げたとおり、あなたはやせ型で妊娠初期ですから、気兼ねなくもっと体重を増やしていいですよ。体の小さい女性にとっては奇妙でしょうが、あなたは赤ちゃんを宿しているのですから、ダイエットをする時期ではありませんね。

P：まあ、もちろんです。

D：ドップラー心拍計で赤ちゃんの心拍音を聞きましょう。すべて正常です。

語句・表現

second trimester：妊娠中期（第2期）
prenatal care：妊婦健診（健康診査）
underweight：体重不足の
heart rate Doppler：ドップラー心拍計

Chapter 17 · 産婦人科

●●● 産婦人科　使える表現

診察

☐ ちょうど妊娠中期に入ったところですね。

❋ You're just entering your second trimester.

☐ 最初のお子さんですか。

❋ Is this your first child?

☐ 腹部を検査したいと思います。いくつか測定の記録を取ります。

❋ I'd like to examine your belly. I'm going to record some measurements.

☐ ドップラー心拍計で赤ちゃんの心音を聞きましょう。

❋ Let's listen to the baby's heart rate with the heart rate Doppler.

☐ 16週目の検診で来院される際に、子宮底長を測ります。これは恥骨と子宮の頂点の間の長さのことです。

When you come in for your 16-week check-up, we'll measure your fundal height. It's the distance between your pubic bone and the top of your uterus.

▶ fundal height：子宮底長　　pubic bone：恥骨　　uterus：子宮

帝王切開

☐ 双子を妊娠しているので、帝王切開の予約を入れます。

Because you're carrying twins, we're going to schedule a caesarean section.

▶ caesarean section [C-section]：帝王切開

☐ 私たちの経験では、帝王切開は赤ちゃんにとってより安全な方法だと思います。

In our practice, we believe a caesarean is a safer bet for the babies.

☐ ますます多くの女性が双子を昔ながらの普通分娩で出産するようになっていることは知っていますが、約40%の割合で、結局は帝王切開で出産しています。

I know that there are more and more women delivering twins the traditional way of vaginal births, but in about 40% of the cases they end up having a C-section.

▶ vaginal birth：普通分娩

2 分娩 ●●● Childbirth

出産についての説明

- **N** 出産について何か質問はありますか。
  Do you have any questions about the delivery?
  - **Pt.** なぜ入院期間がこんなに長いのか気になります。イギリスではたいてい2日ほどですが、先生からは4、5日ほどと伺っています。
    I'm curious why the hospital stay is so long. It's usually about two days in the U.K. and your information talks about four to five days.

- 習慣が非常に異なっているのはよくわかりますが、初産婦さんですから、傷を治し、当院の専門家から育児のコツを学ぶ時間がとれることは実際ありがたく思うかもしれませんよ。
  I realize that the custom is quite different; but as a first time mother, you may really appreciate the time to heal and get nursing tips from the experts here.
  - ▶ **heal**：（一般的に）外傷を治す
  - cf. **cure** ＝病気・けがなどを治してもとの健康な状態に戻す
  - **remedy** ＝薬や特別な方法を用いて病状・苦痛をいやす

- 時に、赤ちゃんは授乳を嫌がることがあります。長く入院していただくと、私たちは起こり得るどんな問題点でも見つけられるかもしれません。
  Sometimes babies are reluctant to nurse. Having you in the hospital longer gives us a chance to catch any possible wrinkles.
  - ▶ **wrinkle**：欠点

- すべての妊婦さんには、「母子手帳」と呼ばれる冊子が最寄りの市・区役所に用意されています。これは手引書の一種です。
  There's a booklet that all expectant mothers get from their city or ward office called a "boshitecho." This is a kind of handbook.

- 妊娠したことを登録すると、役所からこうした教育とモニター用ツールが配布されます。
  You register your pregnancy and they give you this as a kind of educational and monitoring tool.

Chapter 18 - 泌尿器科

1 膀胱炎 ●●● Cystitis

泌尿器科の Dr. Uchida の診察室に排尿のトラブルを抱えた女性がやって来ました。排尿のトラブルは日常生活に直接影響を及ぼします。

Dr. What seems to be the problem?

Pt. I'm experiencing a pain just above my groin.

Dr. Any changes in urination?

Pt. Yes, I feel a strong persistent urge and lately I think my urine looks bright pink.

Dr. Are you noticing any odor?

Pt. Now that you mention it, it smells stronger than before.

Dr. Have you ever had any of these symptoms before?

Pt. No, I don't think so.

Dr. You've mentioned all the typical symptoms of cystitis.

Pt. Cystitis?

Dr. Cystitis is a UTI, a urinary tract infection in your bladder.

Pt. Do you know what causes it?

Dr. It's usually caused by E. coli bacteria.

Pt. E. coli? I don't understand. How was I exposed to that?

Dr. This type of bacteria lives in the intestines of all warm-blooded animals, including people. The problem is most likely that this somehow got into your urine. This is sometimes transmitted sexually, but even if you are not sexually active, women are at risk because of the short distance from the anus to the urethra and from the urethral opening to the bladder.

1 膀胱炎 ●●● Cystitis

訳

D：どうなさいましたか。

P：ちょうど足の付け根の上に痛みを感じています。

D：排尿に何か変化はありますか。

P：はい、絶えず強い尿意があり、最近尿が明るいピンク色のように思えます。

D：においで何か気がつかれましたか。

P：言われてみれば、以前よりにおいが強くなっています。

D：以前、これらの症状になったことはありますか。

P：いいえ、ないと思います。

D：あなたのお話には膀胱炎のあらゆる典型的な症状が含まれています。

P：膀胱炎ですか。

D：膀胱炎は、膀胱内のUTI（尿路感染症）のことです。

P：何が原因か先生はご存知ですか。

D：通常、病原性大腸菌が原因です。

P：大腸菌ですか。わかりません。私はそれにどうやって接触したのでしょう。

D：この種の大腸菌は、人間を含むあらゆる温血動物の腸内に生息します。問題はこれが何らかの原因であなたの尿に入り込んだ可能性があるということです。これは性的に感染する場合がありますが、あなたが性的な行為をなさっていない場合でも、女性は、肛門から尿道まで、および尿道口から膀胱までの距離が短いためにリスクがあるのです。

語句・表現

groin：足の付け根、鼠径部
urination：排尿
odor：におい
UTI (urinary tract infection)：尿路感染症
bladder：膀胱
E. coli bacteria：病原性大腸菌
warm-blooded：温血の、定温の
transmit：感染する
anus：肛門
urethra：尿道

Chapter 18 泌尿器科

●●● 泌尿器科　使える表現

症状をたずねる

☐ **Dr.** 今日はどうなさいましたか。
What brings you here today?
Pt. 排尿時に焼け付くような感覚があります。
I have a burning sensation when I urinate.
▶ burning sensation：焼け付くような感覚

☐ **Dr.** 症状を説明していただけますか。
Could you describe it for me?
Pt. トイレに頻繁に行っていますが、1回の量が少ないのです。
I'm going to the bathroom frequently, but the amount is small each time.

☐ **Dr.** においで何か気がつかれましたか。
❀ Are you noticing any odor?
Pt. 言われてみれば、以前よりにおいが強くなっています。
❀ Now that you mention it, it smells stronger than before.

☐ **Dr.** あなたの尿は、赤ですか、ピンクですか、それともコーラのような色ですか。
Have you noticed that your urine is red, pink or cola-colored?
Pt. 私の尿は赤みを帯びた色です。
My urine looks reddish.

診断

☐ あなたのお話には膀胱炎のあらゆる典型的な症状が含まれています。
❀ You've mentioned all the typical symptoms of cystitis.

☐ 検査結果があらゆる典型的な膀胱炎の症状を示しています。
Your test results indicate all the typical symptoms of cystitis.

☐ 膀胱炎は、膀胱内のUTI（尿路感染症）のことです。
❀ Cystitis is a UTI, a urinary tract infection in your bladder.

☐ 通常、病原性大腸菌が原因です。
❀ It's usually caused by E. coli bacteria.

1 膀胱炎 ●●● Cystitis

- [ ] 1回の排尿量の少なさは、尿路感染症の症状が考えられます。

    Passing small amounts of urine at a time may be a symptom of a urinary tract infection.

- [ ] 尿路感染症の原因について気にするのはやめましょう。

    Let's not concern ourselves with what caused the urinary tract infection.

検査・処置

- [ ] あなたは頻繁に感染症を起こされているので、あなたの尿を培養したいと思います。

    You've had frequent infections so I want to culture your urine.
    - culture：〜を培養する

- [ ] 培養した尿を観察したいと思います。朝一番の尿のサンプルを取っていただき、それを持ってきてください。

    I'd like to follow up with a urine culture. I'll need you to collect a sample of your first urination of the morning and bring it back in.

- [ ] 感染症が頻発しているので、尿路に異常があるかどうかをチェックしたいと思います。造影剤を使ったCTスキャンを行います。

    Because of the frequent infections, I'd like to check for a possible abnormality in your urinary tract. I'd like to do a CT scan with contrast dye.
    - abnormality：異常な状態　　contrast dye：造影剤

- [ ] 膀胱鏡検査の予定を決めたいと思います。今日、新しい尿サンプルを提出してください。検査の前後に抗生物質を服用していただきます。

    I'd like to schedule you for cystoscopy. I'd like to get a new urine sample today. I want you to take antibiotics before and after the test.
    - cystoscopy：膀胱鏡検査　　take antibiotics：抗生物質を服用する

- [ ] あなたの服用している薬をもう一度確認させてください。長く使うと出血の危険性が増えますので。

    I want to review your medications again. There's an increased risk of bleeding.

Chapter 18 - 泌尿器科

2 前立腺肥大 ●●● Enlarged Prostate

泌尿器科のDr. Unoのところに、下腹部に痛みを抱えた男性患者が訪れています。

Pt. I told my regular doctor about this pain I've been having in my abdomen and he sent me to see you.

Dr. Is it tender here?

Pt. OW … Yes!

Dr. Have you noticed anything else unusual besides the pain?

Pt. I've been going to the bathroom a lot and it seems darker than usual.

Dr. Would you lie down for me, please? I'd like to check your lower abdomen. Yes, your bladder feels distended to me. I'd like to do a rectal exam to see if your prostate is enlarged.

Pt. If there's a problem with my bladder, why do I need a prostate exam?

Dr. This exam will tell us a lot ... Just as I suspected ... Your prostate is enlarged. It is likely that you have bladder stones. An enlarged prostate is one of the leading causes of bladder stones. You're 55, and an enlarged prostate is often the disease that men of your age present with when they have bladder stones. I'd like to send you to the radiology department for some X-rays. I'd also like to get a urine sample. Some stones are not visible with conventional X-rays. We want to do a spiral CT-scan to get a better look at what's going on.

語句・表現

prostate：前立腺
abdomen：腹部
distended：膨らんだ、膨張した
rectal exam：直腸検査
bladder stone：膀胱結石
radiology department：放射線科

2　前立腺肥大　●●● Enlarged Prostate

訳

P：かかりつけの医師に私が腹部にずっと抱えているこの痛みについて相談したところ、先生の診察を受けるよう紹介されました。

D：ここを触ると痛いですか。

P：いたっ、はい。

D：痛みの他に何かいつもと違う点には気づかれましたか。

P：私はトイレに頻繁に行っており、尿の色がいつもより濃いようです。

D：横になっていただけますか。下腹部を検査します。ええ、膀胱が膨らんでいるのが触ってわかります。前立腺肥大を確認するため直腸検査を行います。

P：膀胱に問題があると、どうして私は前立腺の検査を受ける必要があるのですか。

D：検査はたくさんのことを示しています。やはり、あなたの前立腺は肥大しています。膀胱結石だと思われます。前立腺肥大は、膀胱結石を引き起こす主要原因の一つです。あなたは55歳ですが、前立腺肥大は、あなたの年代の男性が膀胱結石を発症したときによく見られる疾患なのです。X線写真を撮りに放射線科に行っていただきたいと思います。尿サンプルも提出してください。従来型のX線写真では見えにくい石があります。何が起きているのかもっとよく見えるように、スパイラルCTスキャンを行いたいと思います。

雑学
Spiral CT（スパイラルCT, 螺旋CT）

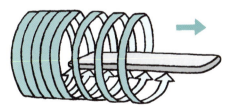

スパイラル（螺旋）CTが登場したのは1989年のことです。**Helical CT**（ヘリカルCT）とも言います。最大の特徴はその撮影方法で、X線をらせん状に照射させながら撮影することで、途切れずに人体を撮影することで、撮影時間の短縮と撮影距離の延長に大きく貢献しました。

泌尿器科　使える表現

症状をたずねる

☐ ここを触ると痛いですか。
- Is it tender here?

☐ **Dr.** あなたが最後に前立腺検査を行ったのはいつでしたか。
- When was the last time you had a prostate exam?

Pt. 2、3年前です。
- A few years ago.

☐ 痛みの他に何かいつもと違う点には気づかれましたか。
- Have you noticed anything else unusual besides the pain?

検査

☐ 前立腺検査を行いたいと思います。
- I'd like to do a prostate exam.

☐ 私はあなたの前立腺のサイズと質感に懸念があります。PSA（前立腺特異抗原）と呼ばれる血液検査を予約しましょう。
- I'm concerned about the size and texture of your prostate. I'm ordering a blood test called PSA, prostate-specific antigen.

☐ 血流中のPSAの数値が高い場合は、感染症やことによるとがんを考慮することになるかもしれません。
- If there's a high amount of PSA in your bloodstream, we could be looking at an infection or possibly cancer.

☐ **Dr.** 前立腺をより詳しく評価するため経直腸超音波検査を行いたいと思います。
- I'd like to do transrectal ultrasound to evaluate your prostate further.

Pt. もう少し詳しく説明していただけますか。
- Could you explain that a bit more?

Dr. もちろんです。この検査ではあなたの直腸に小さなプローブ（探触子）を挿入します。このプローブは音波によってあなたの前立腺の画像を作成します。
- Sure. It involves inserting a small probe in your rectum, that uses sound waves to create a picture of your prostate gland.

▶ transrectal ultrasound：経直腸超音波

☐ 実施した検査があなたの前立腺がんを示唆していることを懸念しています。前立腺生検を行いたいと思います。

I'm concerned that the tests we've conducted indicate you have prostate cancer. I'd like to do a prostate biopsy.

▶ prostate biopsy：前立腺生検

診断

☐ あなたの前立腺は肥大しています。膀胱結石だと思われます。

✤ Your prostate is enlarged. It is likely that you have bladder stones.

☐ 前立腺肥大は、膀胱結石を引き起こす主要原因の一つです。

✤ An enlarged prostate is one of the leading causes of bladder stones.

☐ 検査室ががん細胞を分析したところ、これはステージ1、グリソンスコア2であると判断しました。これは穏やかながんを意味し、狭い範囲に限局しています。

The laboratory analyzed the cancer cells and has determined that this is stage 1 and is a Gleason score of 2, which means this is a nonaggressive cancer, confined to a small area.

▶ Gleason score：グリソンスコア　＊がんの悪性度を示す。

☐ 検査室の結果によると、これはステージ4の前立腺がんです。直ちに化学療法を始めることをお勧めします。

According to the lab results, this is stage 4 prostate cancer. I'm going to recommend that you start chemotherapy right away.

▶ chemotherapy：化学療法

☐ あなたの膀胱には明らかに石があります。小さな石一つであれば、患者さんが大量の水を飲んで、ご自分でそれを流せることがあるのですが、あなたの石はそうではありません。

There are definitely stones in your bladder. Sometimes, if there's one small stone, the patient can drink a lot of water and flush it out himself, but that's not the case here.

Chapter 19 - 形成外科

1　顔面神経麻痺　●●● Facial Paralysis

形成外科のDr. Watanabeは、自分の顔面に異変を見つけて、あわてて診察にやって来た患者から話を聞いています。

Dr. I see what appears to be a facial droop on the left side. When did this start?

Pt. Just yesterday.

Dr. Have you noticed any other symptoms?

Pt. Actually, it hurts behind my ear, I've been drooling, and my breakfast didn't taste very good today. Oh, and my eyes are dry.

Dr. Let me see how you perform a few tasks. Please close your eyes.

Pt. Okay. (Patient closes eyes)

Dr. Go ahead and open your eyes. Could you blink for me? All right, Lift your right eyebrow. Good … now lift your left eyebrow … smile with your teeth showing … now, frown ….

I'm going to order an EMG, a nerve conduction study, which the nurse will explain to you later. I think you have Bell's palsy, which is a type of facial paralysis. It can often be temporary, which is the good news, but we want to be proactive and see if we can push it to run its course faster. I'm going to prescribe medication and give you eye drops.

Pt. I see. When do I need to come back in and see you?

Dr. The nurse will schedule the nerve conduction study and then call you to make an appointment after I've had a look at that. I'm going to prescribe two weeks' worth of medication.

Pt. Thank you very much.

1 顔面神経麻痺　Facial Paralysis

訳

D：あなたの顔の左側に下垂が現れているのがわかります。この症状はいつ始まりましたか。

P：昨日始まったばかりです。

D：何か他の症状には気づかれましたか。

P：実は、耳の後ろが痛み、いつもよだれが出ますし、今日の朝食はあまりおいしく感じませんでした。それから、目が乾燥しています。

D：いくつか、私の指示に従って動かせるかどうか見せてください。目を閉じてください。

P：わかりました。（患者が目を閉じる）

D：そのまま続けて、それから目を開けてください。私に向かってまばたきをしていただけますか。結構です。右の眉を上げてください。結構ですよ。…では、左の眉を上げてください。歯を見せて笑ってください。次は眉をひそめてください。

EMG（筋電図検査）、すなわち神経伝導検査を手配しましょう。看護師が後ほど説明いたします。あなたの症状は顔面神経麻痺の一種のベル麻痺だと思います。ベル麻痺は、これは朗報ですが、一時的なものであることが多く、私たちは積極的に、自然治癒の方向により早く向かえるかやってみたいと思います。薬を処方して、目薬をお出ししましょう。

P：わかりました。いつ再診に来ればよいでしょうか。

D：看護師が神経伝導検査の予約を入れ、それから私が検査結果を拝見した後であなたに予約を取るための電話をいたします。2週間分の薬を処方しましょう。

P：ありがとうございます。

語句・表現

facial droop：顔面下垂
drool：よだれを垂らす
blink：まばたきをする
frown：眉をひそめる、顔をしかめる
EMG：筋電図検査
nerve conduction study：神経伝導検査
proactive：積極的な、前向きな
run its course：自然に治癒する

形成外科　使える表現

症状をたずねる

☐ 顔の左側に下垂が現れているのがわかります。

❈ I see what appears to be a facial droop on the left side.

☐ 目を閉じ続けていることが困難であり、それで寝付けないとのことですね。

It says that you're having trouble keeping your eye closed, so it must be hard to fall asleep.

☐ 今までに顔の筋肉がゆがんだり、引きつったことはありますか。

Have you ever had a twisting or pulling feeling in your face?

☐ あなたの顔面下垂はいつ始まりましたか。

When did your facial droop start?

☐ 他の症状で何か気がついたことはありますか。

❈ Have you noticed any other symptoms?

診断

☐ あなたは、顔面神経麻痺の一種のベル麻痺だと思います。

❈ I think you have Bell's palsy, which is a type of facial paralysis.

☐ 直ちに顔面麻痺を発見し、コルチコステロイド剤を使った治療を開始しましたので、予後は良好です。

Since we caught the facial paralysis right away and began treating it with corticosteroids, the prognosis is good.

▶ corticosteroids：コルチコステロイド剤　　prognosis：予後

治療・助言

☐ **Dr.** 規則的に手を使ってまばたきをしていただきたいと思います。

I want you to manually blink your eye regularly.

Pt. 「手を使ってまばたきをする」とはどういう意味ですか。

What do you mean by "manually blink" my eye?

Dr. 目に乾いている感じを覚えた時にはいつでも、指の背を使ってまぶたを上下に動かしてください。

1 顔面神経麻痺 ●●● Facial Paralysis

Whenever your eye feels dry, use the back of your finger to move your eyelid up and down.
> blink one's eye：まばたきをする

☐ 濃い軟膏タイプの潤滑点眼薬と眼帯の使用を試していただきましょう。効き目があるはずです。

Let's try having you apply a thick eye lubricant ointment and a pirate's patch. That should do the trick.
> lubricant：潤滑油
> eye lubricant ointment：潤滑点眼薬 ＊潤滑油を含み通常の目薬よりも濃い点眼薬。
> pirate's patch：アイパッチ、眼帯
> do the trick：効き目がある

☐ **Dr.** 水泳用のゴーグルか目の周りに巻きつけるタイプのサングラスを持っていらっしゃいますか。

Do you happen to have swimming goggles or wraparound sunglasses?

Pt. はい、いくつか水泳用ゴーグルを持っています。
Yes, I do have some swim goggles.

Dr. それを夜に着用してみてください。これが「加湿器」の役目を果たします。
I'd like you to try wearing them in the evening. This will create a "moisture chamber."
> moisture chamber：加湿器

☐ あなたに当病院の眼科医を紹介します。眼科医が特別に目を保護するものが必要かどうかを判断してくれるでしょう。

I'm going to refer you to the ophthalmologist here at the hospital. She can decide whether you need special protective eye gear.

☐ **Dr.** まぶたにつける重りを処方します。
I'm prescribing eyelid weights for you.

Pt. それはどういった働きをするのですか。
How do they work?

Dr. 毎朝、まぶたのま上に1枚貼ってください。重りはあなたがよりうまくまばたきできるよう手助けします。

You attach one just above the eyelashes every morning. The weight will help you blink more successfully.

Chapter 20 - 皮膚科

1　皮膚アレルギー　Skin Allergies

Dr. Yoshida の元にひどい湿疹を発症させた患者が駆け込んできました。どうやら日本に来て見慣れない麺を食べたようです。

Dr. Good morning. The chart says you're here because of a rash … whoa … you certainly are broken out everywhere. Have you experienced any trouble breathing?

Pt. No. My skin is just hot to the touch and itchy.

Dr. And did this just start today?

Pt. Yes, right after lunch.

Dr. What was your lunch?

Pt. I tried some brownish Japanese noodles for the first time …

Dr. Soba? You ate buckwheat noodles?

Pt. That's it!

Dr. We can do some allergy testing after we clear this up, but buckwheat is a known allergen. It's a safe bet that your hives were caused by that. In addition to the noodles, buckwheat flour is sometimes used in other Japanese cooking, so you should make sure that what you're eating is buckwheat-free.

Pt. Okay.

Dr. I'm going to give you two prescriptions. One is for a salve that should help with the itching and the healing of your skin. The other is a non-drowsy antihistamine. I'm going to put you on a relatively high dose of this to see if we can clear up your hives and get the allergen out of your system. Feel free to cut down or stop the antihistamine completely once the symptoms stop. If it doesn't clear up in a few days, I want you to come back in.

1 皮膚アレルギー ●●● Skin Allergies

訳

D：おはようございます。このカルテには、あなたは湿疹のためにここへいらしたとありますが、ああ、確かにあらゆるところ出ていますね。呼吸に何かトラブルを経験したことはありますか。

P：いいえ。触ると熱くてかゆいだけです。

D：それで、これは今日始まったのですか。

P：はい、昼食の直後に。

D：昼食は何でしたか。

P：私は、茶色っぽい日本製の麺を初めて食べてみました。

D：ソバですか。ソバ粉の麺を食べたのですか。

P：それが私が食べたものです。

D：この発疹をきれいにしたあと、アレルギー検査をすることができますが、ソバはアレルギー誘発物質として知られています。あなたのじんましんはそれが原因であることは間違いありません。麺に加えて、ソバ粉は他の和食に使われることがありますので、あなたは食べているものがソバを含んでいないことを確かめてください。

P：わかりました。

D：二つの処方薬をお渡しします。一つは皮膚のかゆみを抑えて治癒を促す軟膏です。もう一つは眠くならない抗ヒスタミン剤です。じんましんをきれいにして、身体からアレルギー誘発物質を取り除くかどうかを確認するために、比較的多量の投与を行うつもりです。その症状が収まったら、抗ヒスタミン剤を減らすか完全にやめていただいて構いません。数日間投与しても症状がなくならない場合は、また診察にいらしてください。

語句・表現

rash：湿疹
break out 〜：〜を発生する
buckwheat noodle：ソバ
clear up 〜：（湿疹など）をきれいにする
It is a safe bet that ...：間違いなく…である

hives：じんましん
salve：軟膏
non-drowsy：眠くならない
antihistamine：抗ヒスタミン剤

皮膚科　使える表現

症状をたずねる

☐ 発疹がありますか。
Do you have a rash? / Do you have hives?

☐ 発疹の場所はどこですか。
Where is the rash on your body?

☐ 他の部位へ広がっていますか。
Has it spread to anywhere else?

☐ かゆみがありますか。
Does it feel itchy?

☐ 他に徴候や症状がありますか。
Do you have any other signs or symptoms?

☐ 呼吸に何かトラブルを経験したことはありますか。
Have you experienced any trouble breathing?

☐ これまでにアレルギー反応を起こしたことがありますか。
Have you ever had any allergic reactions?

診断

☐ ソバはアレルギー誘発物質として知られています。あなたのじんましんはそれが原因であることは間違いありません。
Buckwheat is a known allergen. It's a safe bet that your hives were caused by that.

☐ この検査結果によると、どうもあなたは魚のアレルギーではないようです。おそらく、寄生虫アレルギーではないかと思われます。
Based on this test, you don't seem to be allergic to fish. I suspect it could be a parasite allergy.

☐ 私たちが行ったすべての検査の結果は陰性でした。
Every test we've run has been negative.

処置・処方

☐ 一つは皮膚のかゆみを抑えて治癒を促す軟膏です。もう一つは眠くならない抗ヒスタミン剤です。

❋ One is for a salve that should help with the itching and the healing of your skin. The other is a non-drowsy antihistamine.

☐ あなたが受けている抗ヒスタミン剤の投薬計画は少し効果を示しているようですので、それを継続したいと思います。

It seems you've been doing a little better on the regimen of antihistamines you've been on, so I'd like you to keep that up.

▶ regimen：投薬計画

☐ 抗ヒスタミン薬の投与量をもっと増やす必要がありそうです。

Perhaps we need to try you at a higher dose of the antihistamines.

☐ その症状が収まったら、抗ヒスタミン剤を減らすか完全にやめていただいて構いません。

❋ Feel free to cut down or stop the antihistamine completely once the symptoms stop.

☐ **Pt.** アレルギー薬はかなりよく効いていると思いますが、実はまだ頭皮がかゆいという問題があります。

I think the allergy pills are working pretty well, but I'm actually still having a problem with my scalp being itchy.

Dr. 特に頭皮用のものを処方します。小さな回転塗布式のもので、局所ステロイドを含んでいます。頭のかゆい所にたっぷりと使ってください。

I'm going to prescribe something specifically for your scalp. It's a little roll-on that contains a topical steroid. Use it generously on the itchy spots on your head.

▶ roll-on：回転塗布式の　　topical steroid：局所ステロイド

☐ **Pt.** 美容師から薬用シャンプーを入手しましたが、まだ頭皮にかゆみがあります。

I got a medicated shampoo from the hairdresser, but my scalp still itches.

Dr. 薬用シャンプーと呼ばれるシャンプーのほとんどは、あまり強い効き目はないので、今だにかゆみがあっても驚くことではありません。

Most of the so-called medicated shampoos are not very strong, so it isn't surprising that you're still itchy.

Chapter 20 - 皮膚科

2 できもの ... Skin Tumors

皮膚科の Dr. Yoshida の診察室にやって来た患者は以前からあった胸の下のできものが痛みを伴うようになってきたようです。

Dr. Good morning. What seems to be the trouble today?

Pt. I have this reddish growth right below my breast. I've had it for a while, but lately, it seems to be getting irritated when I get dressed and undressed.

Dr. Let's have a look. I see … It's a skin tag. I think we should try freezing this off with liquid nitrogen. It will probably require a few treatments, but I believe we can deal with it easily this way.

Pt. Sounds good.

(Pause)

Dr. All right. Could you hold your shirt up? I also want you to look away. This is going to feel cold.

Pt. Ah…it is cold!

Dr. Give it a second before you put your shirt back down. I suspect this is going to ooze, so you may find some reddish-brown spots on your clothes. Let's make an appointment for you to have another treatment next week.

Pt. You said a few treatments. Is that like three or four?

Dr. That's about how long it takes in my experience, but individuals differ. The last patient I treated with liquid nitrogen for something about this size saw it completely fall off after the third treatment.

語句・表現

reddish growth：赤みを帯びた
irritated：ひりひりする
skin tag：スキン・タグ、軟性線維腫
liquid nitrogen：液体窒素
look away：目をそらす
ooze：にじみ出る

訳

D：おはようございます。今日はどうなさいましたか。

P：胸のすぐ下に、この赤みを帯びたできものがあります。しばらくこれがあるのですが、最近服を脱ぎ着するときにひりひりするように思います。

D：それでは拝見します。なるほど…これはスキン・タッグ（軟性線維腫）です。液体窒素を使って凍らせて取りましょう。何回か治療が必要となるでしょうが、この方法で容易に対処できると思います。

P：それはいいですね。（中断）

D：用意できました。シャツを持ち上げていただけますか。目もそらしていただきたいと思います。大変に冷たく感じますよ。

P：あー、冷たい！

D：シャツを下ろすのを少し待ってください。これ（液体窒素）がにじみ出るかもしれませんので、服に赤みがかった茶色のしみが付くかもしれません。来週の次回の治療のために、予約を取りましょう。

P：何回かの治療とのことですね。それは3、4回といった感じでしょうか。

D：私の経験ではそれくらいですが、個人差があります。私がこのくらいの大きさのもの（できもの）に液体窒素療法を行った直近の患者さんは、3回目の治療後に完全な除去を確認しました。

雑学
メラノーマ（黒色腫）の見分け方

メラノーマは一見ほくろと勘違いされることが多いのですが、皮膚がんの中でも非常に悪性度が高いことで知られています。英語には、患者がメラノーマを確認するときに覚えておくシステムがあります。これはABCDEシステムと呼ばれています。

A（**asymmetry** 非対称）：できものの中央に線を描いてみて、右と左で形状が同じになっていない。

B（**borders** ヘリ・縁）：初期のメラノーマに見られ、ヘリ・縁が一定でなくでこぼこしている。

C（**color** 色）：単色でなくさまざまな色調が見られる。

D（**diameter** 直径）：直径が消しゴム付きの鉛筆の消しゴムより大きい。

E（**evolving** 発達）：大きさ、形状、色などに変化が認められる。さらに、出血、痛み、かゆみを伴うと、メラノーマの前兆の可能性がある。

皮膚科　使える表現

症状をたずねる

- **Dr.** 最初に皮膚にこのできものが現れたのはいつですか。
  When did this mark on your skin first appear?
- **Pt.** 数ケ月前に気が付きました。
  I noticed it a few months ago.

- **Dr.** 大きさや形に何か変化はありますか。
  Has there been any change in size or shape?
- **Pt.** 最初に気がついた時よりも大きくなっていると思います。
  I think it's bigger than when I first noticed it.

- **Dr.** 何か痛み、かゆみ、あるいは出血はありますか。
  Are you aware of any pain, itching or bleeding with it?
- **Pt.** 最近かゆみがあります。
  It's been itchy lately.

- あなたの体のどこかにこのようなあざ・しみを見つけたことがありますか。
  Have you seen spots like this anywhere else on your body?

- 繰り返し日焼けをしたことがありますか。
  Have you had repeated sunburns?

診断・治療

- これはスキン・タッグです。液体窒素を使って凍らせて取りましょう。
- ❂ It's a skin tag. I think we should try freezing this off with liquid nitrogen.

- 何回か治療が必要となるでしょうが、この方法で容易に対処できると思います。
- ❂ It will probably require a few treatments, but I think we can deal with it easily this way.

- 腫瘍は悪性です。病状から見て、あなたに最初にしていただきたいことは、腫瘍を切除する手術の予定を入れることです。
  The tumor is malignant. Based on the pathology, the first thing I'd like to do is schedule surgery to excise it.

2 できもの ●●● Skin Tumors

▶ malignant：悪性の　　pathology：病理、病状
excise：（身体から）～を切除（摘出）する

☐ この腫瘍が再発したものなので、モーズ手術を行いたいと思います。

Because this tumor has recurred, we'd like to treat it with Mohs surgery.

☐ モーズ手術は、皮膚を一層ごとに切りはがして、顕微鏡の下で、層に異常をきたしている細胞が検出されない層に到達するまで、顕微鏡で確認する手術です。

Mohs surgery is a procedure where we excise the skin layer by layer, examining it under a microscope until we get to a layer without abnormal cells.

☐ 何か見過ごしていないことを確認するためにPETスキャン検査を入れるつもりです。

I am going to order a PET scan to make sure that we haven't missed anything.

▶ PET scan (positron-emission tomography scan)：放射断層撮影法スキャン

☐ 2ラウンドの化学療法を終え、希望通りの治療効果が腫瘍に現れていることを確認したら、もう一つPETスキャンを行います。

We'll also do another PET scan after you finish two rounds of chemotherapy to see if the tumor is responding to treatment as hoped.

☐ 非ホジキンリンパ腫（NHL）向けの化学療法薬は心臓や肺に影響を及ぼす傾向があるので、投与する前に、心臓と肺の機能を広範囲にわたってテストしたいと思います。

The chemotherapy drugs used for NHL tend to affect the heart and lungs, so we want to test your heart and lung function extensively, before starting chemo.

▶ chemo：chemotherapy（化学療法）の略

☐ 病状が進行しているため、併用療法を試みたいと思います。化学療法および免疫療法だけでなく、経口ステロイドを併用していただきます。

Because the disease is spreading, we want to try a combination therapy. You'll get immunotherapy along with chemotherapy treatments, as well as an oral steroid.

▶ combination therapy：併用療法　　immunotherapy：免疫療法

3 抜け毛 ●●● Hair Loss

Chapter 20 - 皮膚科

皮膚科の Dr. Yoshida は抜け毛を気にして訪れた患者を診察しますが、どうやら抜け毛以上に気になる症状があるようです。

Dr. I see something on your arm. Hmm, the margins of the lesion are crusty.

Pt. I've been losing a lot of hair recently. See how my hairline is receded on the left side. All of that hair has fallen out recently.

Dr. You only mentioned the hair loss when you checked in today, but I am concerned about it in conjunction with the lesion on your arm. Do you have any sores anywhere else?

Pt. There's something on the inside of my nose too …

Dr. Let me have a look. (pause) First, I want to get a complete blood count (CBC) and an antinuclear antibody (ANA) test. Then, I'll take a urine sample. When we get all this, we'll send you to the Radiology Department for a chest X-ray.

Pt. All right.

Dr. I think you may have some form of lupus. We'll take a kidney biopsy to confirm, but I want to use the least invasive methods we have. I have to tell you that the shape and crusty nature of the lesions make me think that it may be a foregone conclusion that we are, in fact, dealing with lupus here.

Pt. I've heard that lupus is very serious.

Dr. Unfortunately, we don't have as many treatment options for autoimmune disorders as we'd like, but there are many new studies. One theory is that people with lupus create too many antibodies and these antibodies attack healthy cells. This sort of research is very new, but I believe it will help us create better treatments.

3 抜け毛 ●●● Hair Loss

訳

D：腕に何かありますね。うーむ、皮膚の病斑の周辺部が硬いですね。

P：最近、髪の毛がたくさん抜けています。左側の髪の生え際が後退しているのがおわかりでしょう。この部分の髪の毛は全部、最近抜け落ちたのです。

D：受付では、抜け毛のことだけをお話になりましたが、それと腕の病斑との関連が気になります。どこか他の部分に痛みはありますか。

P：鼻の中にも痛むところがあります。

D：ちょっと見せてください。(中断) まず、全血算定（CBC）と抗核抗体（ANA）検査を行います。その上で、尿サンプルを取りましょう。すべてを終えたら、レントゲンを撮りに、放射線科へ行っていただきます。

P：わかりました。

D：あなたの症状は、何らかの狼瘡（ろうそう）の類かと思われます。確認のため、腎生検を行いますが、侵襲性の最も低い方法を使います。その皮膚の損傷の形状と固さの性質から、これは実際、当院で狼瘡として対応している症状だと言わざるを得ません。

P：狼瘡はとても深刻だと聞きましたが。

D：残念ながら、自己免疫疾患の治療法の選択肢は、望むほど多くはありませんが、新しい研究が数多くあります。ある理論は狼瘡の患者さんは抗体を過度に作り出し、この抗体が健康な細胞を攻撃しているというものです。これは新しい研究の鍵になる事実で、これがよりよい治療をするのに役立つと信じています。

語句・表現

margins：縁、周縁部
lesion：(皮膚の) 損傷、病気
crusty：堅い皮のある、皮殻質の
complete blood count (CBC)：全血算定
antinuclear antibody (ANA)：抗核抗体
lupus：狼瘡、ループス
＊種々の皮膚のびらんや疾患を特徴とする。
least invasive：最小限に侵襲性の
foregone conclusion：当然の結果、予測できる結末
autoimmune disorders：自己免疫疾患

Chapter 20 皮膚科

●●● 皮膚科　使える表現

症状をたずねる

□ 頭髪に変化がありましたか。
Have you noticed any change in your hair?

□ 最近ひどい抜け毛がありましたか。
Have you recently noticed any excessive hair loss?

□ 何か脱毛の原因として考えられることはありますか。
What do you think is causing your hair loss?

□ どれくらいの頻度で髪を洗いますか。
How often do you wash your hair?

□ どこか他の部分に痛みはありますか。
❈ Do you have any sores anywhere else?

診断

□ あなたの頭皮には何も炎症を起こしている部分はどこにも見当たりません。
I don't see any irritated areas on your scalp.

□ 1日に50から100本の間で髪の毛が抜けるのは自然なことです。それ以上抜け落ちるのであれば、それは何らかの病気のサインのことがありますが、ストレスが原因かもしれません。
It's natural to lose between 50 and 100 strands a day. If more than that is falling out, it is can be indicative of some sort of a disease, but, then again, it may be caused by stress.

□ 抜け毛の原因は円形脱毛症ですが、これは極度のストレスからもたらされた可能性があります。
The reason for the hair loss is that you have alopecia areata, which may have been caused by extreme stress.
　▶ alopecia areata：円形脱毛症

□ 円形脱毛症では、体の免疫システムが毛穴にダメージを与えて抜け毛を引き起こします。
Alopecia areata is a condition in which the body's immune system attacks the hair follicles and causes hair loss.
　▶ hair follicles：毛穴

3 抜け毛 ●●● Hair Loss

- [ ] その皮膚の損傷の形状と固さの性質から、これは当院で狼瘡として対応している症状だと言わざるを得ません。

  ❇ I have to tell you that the shape and crusty nature of the lesions make me think that it's foregone conclusion that we are dealing with lupus here.

- [ ] お嬢さんは緊張したり、感情が高ぶった時に髪の毛を引き抜くようです。この症状は抜毛癖と呼ばれます。

  Your daughter seems to pull out her hair when she's dealing with tension or some other strong emotions. This condition is called trichotillomania.
  ▶ trichotillomania：抜毛癖

- [ ] このタイプの抜け毛は休止期脱毛と呼ばれ、ほとんどの場合、やがて治癒します。

  This type of hair loss is called telogen effluvium and it almost always corrects itself over time.
  ▶ telogen effluvium：休止期脱毛

処置・処方

- [ ] 抜け毛用の局所軟膏をお渡ししますが、下の階へ行って血液検査をしていただきたいと思います。あなたの甲状腺に何も問題がないことをダブルチェックすべきだと思います。

  I'm going to give you a topical ointment for the hair loss, but I'd like to send you downstairs for a blood test. I believe that we should double check that you don't have some issue with your thyroid.
  ▶ topical ointment：局所軟膏　　thyroid：甲状腺

- [ ] 甲状腺機能低下も甲状腺機能亢進も、抜け毛の原因となり得るのです。この軟膏を1日に一度塗ってください。

  Both an underactive and an overactive thyroid can cause hair loss. I'd like you to apply this once a day.

- [ ] 非常に強い匂いがありますので、夜に使ってください。

  It has a very strong smell, so you may want to use it at night.

- [ ] この症状は一時的です。悩んだり、頭皮に何か薬を塗る必要はないと思います。

  This situation is temporary. I don't think you need to worry or apply any kind of medication to your scalp.

Chapter 21 - 眼科

1 ドライアイ ●●● Dry Eye Syndrome

眼科のDr. Zaizenの元に、ドライアイ症候群と診断された患者がやってきました。近年、コンピュータの多用によりこの症状の患者が増えています。

Dr. So your former doctor diagnosed you with dry eye syndrome?

Pt. Yes, that's right. I saw a doctor a year ago for DES. I considered LipiFlow treatment, but it wasn't that bad at the time. Now, I'm living in a more urban environment and working on a computer many hours a day.

Dr. I can imagine that you're exposed to more dust in this environment. I'd like to take a closer look at your eyes. Let's have you sit in my chair over here.

Pt. Yes.

Dr. All right, I'm going to do a little test with some drops now. I want to calculate your "tear film break-up time." You probably have had this done before, but I'd like to get my own sense of your condition.

Pt. Sure. (long pause)

Dr. I definitely do see dry patches in both of your eyes. I know of at least one colleague in Tokyo using LipiFlow.

Pt. Really? I spend a lot of time in Tokyo.

Dr. I'd be happy to write you a referral, but why don't we try a more conservative treatment first? We can do a simple treatment now. We'll apply a warm compress to your eyelids and manually express your meibomian glands. Let's move you over to that chair.

Pt. Okay.

1 ドライアイ ●●● Dry Eye Syndrome

訳

D：それで、前の主治医の先生は、あなたをドライアイ症候群と診断されたのですね。

P：はい、そのとおりです。私は1年前にドライアイ症候群で受診しました。LipiFlow治療を検討したのですが、あの当時は、さほど悪化していませんでした。今は、もっと都会の環境で生活していますし、1日の多くの時間を、コンピュータを使って仕事をしています。

D：この環境では、あなたがより多くのほこりにさらされているのは想像できます。あなたの目をもう少し近くで見たいと思います。ここにある私の椅子に座ってください。

P：はい。

D：それでは、今から点眼薬を使ってちょっとした検査を行います。あなたの涙液層破壊時間を測りたいのです。たぶんあなたは、この検査は以前行ったことがあると思いますが、私は自分の判断であなたの状態を把握したいのです。

P：もちろんです。（長い中断）

D：間違いなくあなたの両眼にドライスポットがあります。私はLipiFlowを使っている医師を東京で少なくとも1人知っていますよ。

P：本当ですか。東京にはしょっちゅう行きます。

D：喜んで紹介状を書きますが、まずは、もっと保存療法を行ってみませんか。今、簡単な治療をすることができるのです。まぶたに温かい布をあてがい、マイボーム腺を手で絞り出します。さあ、あちら側の椅子に移動しましょう。

P：わかりました。

語句・表現

LipiFlow：TearScience社が開発した、眼瞼縁を結膜側から温めるとともに圧迫マッサージする方法。

drops：点眼薬

tear film break-up time：涙液層破壊時間

dry patch：ドライスポット（涙膜の薄くなった部分）

conservative treatment：保存療法、対処療法

meibomian glands：マイボーム腺
＊上下のまぶたの内側にあり、目を乾燥から守る脂質がでる分泌腺。

眼科　使える表現

症状をたずねる

☐ 目が乾いている感じですか。
Do your eyes feel dry?

☐ 目やにが出ますか。
Do you have any discharge from your eyes?

☐ 涙がたくさん出ますか。
Do your eyes water a lot?

☐ 目の動きを調節しにくいですか。
Do you have difficulty controlling your eye movements?

☐ 目の疲れがありますか。
Are you experiencing any eyestrain?

検査

☐ もう少し近くで見せてください。瞳を開かせるために、何滴か点眼剤を入れますね。
I'd like to take a closer look. I'm going to put some drops in your eyes to dilate them.
▶ dilate：〜を広げる、拡張させる

☐ 今から点滴薬を使ってちょっとした検査を行います。あなたの涙液層破壊時間を測りたいのです。
❋ I'm going to do a little test with some drops now. I want to calculate your "tear film break-up time."

☐ まぶたを押しますので、違和感があるかもしれません。
I'm going to press on your eyelids, which may feel strange.

☐ それぞれの目に綿棒で少し麻酔薬を塗ってから、まぶたを裏返します。
I'm going to apply a little anesthetic to each eye with a cotton swab and then I'm going to evert your eyelids.
▶ anesthetic：麻酔薬　　apply 〜 with a cotton swab：綿棒で〜を塗る（塗布する）
　 evert：（まぶた・唇など）を裏返す

診断・治療

☐ 間違いなくあなたの両眼にドライスポットがあります。

❋ I definitely do see dry patches in both of your eyes.

☐ 長時間コンピュータに向かったり、スマートフォンを使ったりしたことが、ドライアイを引き起こしています。

Spending so much time at the computer and using a smartphone have been linked to dry eye syndrome.

☐ コンタクトレンズを使用している人はドライアイを患う可能性があります。

Many contact lens users suffer from dry eye syndrome.

☐ あなたは仕事で、1日の大半をコンピュータに向かわなければいけないようですね。当面の間は、人工涙液を処方したいと思います。

It sounds like your job is keeping you at the computer most of the day. I'd like to prescribe artificial tears for the time being.

☐ まぶたに温湿布をあてがい、マイボーム腺を手で絞り出します。

❋ We'll apply a warm compress to your eyelids and manually express your meibomian glands.

☐ コンタクトレンズを着用する1日あたりの時間を減らし、しっかり目の治療計画に従ってください。

You probably need to start wearing your contacts fewer hours a day and follow a tight eye care regimen.
▶ regimen：投薬・治療計画

☐ 追加検査により、眼瞼炎という、まつげの毛根の感染症にかかっていることがわかりました。

Further tests indicate that you have an infection of your eyelash roots called blepharitis.
▶ eyelash root：まつげの毛根　　blepharitis：眼瞼炎

☐ 症状からすると、実はシェーグレン症候群の可能性が考えられます。

Based on your symptoms, I think you might actually have Sjogren's syndrome.

Chapter 21 - 眼科

2 白内障　Cataracts

眼科のDr. Zaizenのもとに次にやって来た患者は、以前よりも物が見えにくくなったと訴えています。

Dr. Would you say that your vision is blurry?

Pt. Yes. It's not as clear as it used to be.

Dr. Do you notice any changes at night?

Pt. Absolutely. It's much harder to see at night. Actually, I stopped driving at night because of this.

Dr. Does light or glare bother you more than it used to?

Pt. Now that you mention it, yes.

Dr. Is there anything else going on with your eyes that comes to mind?

Pt. I don't know if I can describe this well, but it's like colors are a bit faded or yellowed …

Dr. Many patients talk about images seeming yellowed. I know what you mean.

Pt. Oh, and it's a bit harder to read than it used to be.

Dr. Yes, everything you've described, including the yellowing of colors, sounds like typical cataract symptoms.

Pt. Does that mean I need surgery?

Dr. We can sometimes recommend other interventions before surgery, but your symptoms already seem to be affecting your quality of life. I want to do an eye exam, but I think we'll need to think about surgery.

語句・表現

blurry：ぼやける、かすむ
glare：まぶしい光

intervention：治療介入

2 白内障 ●●● Cataracts

訳

D：視界がぼやけるとおっしゃいましたね。

P：はい。以前のようにはっきり見えません。

D：夜に何か変化に気が付きますか。

P：もちろんです。夜はずっと見えにくくなります。実際のところ、このせいで夜の運転をやめました。

D：以前よりも日光あるいはまぶしい光が気になるでしょうか。

P：そう言われてみると、そうです。

D：他に何か目に関して思い浮かぶことはありますか。

P：このことをうまく言葉で表現できるかどうかわかりませんが、色が少しばかり薄くなったり、黄色っぽくなるように見えます。

D：多くの患者さんが黄色く見えるイメージのことをお話しになります。おっしゃっていることがよくわかります。

P：あ、それから以前よりも文字を読むことが少し大変になっています。

D：はい、あなたが言われたことは、黄色く変色することを含めてすべてが、典型的な白内障の症状のように思われます。

P：それは手術が必要だということでしょうか。

D：手術をする前に、別の治療をお勧めすることがありますが、あなたの症状はすでに生活の質に影響を及ぼしているようです。目の検査を行いますが、手術のことを考える必要があると思います。

表現のポイント

患者にはできるだけ専門用語ではなく、わかりやすい表現を使います。

	Professional term(s)	Lay term(s)
視力	visual acuity	vision
水晶体	crystalline lens	lens
混濁	opacity（形容詞）	cloudy

眼科　使える表現

症状をたずねる

☐ 視界がぼやけるとおっしゃいましたね。
❀ Would you say that your vision is blurry?

☐ 視力はどんな具合に悪化しているのでしょうか。
How has your vision been getting worse?

☐ 夜に何か変化に気が付きますか。
❀ Do you notice any changes at night?

☐ 物が二重に見える問題を抱えていると書いていらっしゃるのですね。
I see that you wrote down that you are having issues with double vision.

☐ 今までに目の手術を受けたことはありますか。
Have you ever had eye surgery before?

診察

☐ 目を見せてください。水晶体が混濁していますね。
Let me take a look at your eyes ... Your lenses are cloudy.

☐ 目の精密検査を行う必要があります。
We need to do a thorough eye exam.

☐ あなたの瞳を広げるためにこれから点眼をします。その後は、点眼薬が効き始めるまで待合室にお戻りいただきます。
We're going to put some drops in your eyes to dilate them. After that, I'll ask you to step back into the waiting area until they start to take effect.

▶ dilate：〜を拡張する、広げる

診断・治療

☐ ほとんどの白内障は加齢と関わりがあります。年配の方に非常によく見られる症状です。

Most cataracts are related to aging. Cataracts are very common in older people.

☐ まだ手術の必要はないと思います。まず眼鏡の度数を変え、それで改善するか様子を見ましょう。

I don't think you need surgery yet. First, let's try changing the prescription of your glasses and see if that works for you.

☐ 検査結果とあなたからの説明に基づいて、白内障の手術を予定したいと思います。今回は、片方の目だけを手術しようと思います。

Based on the tests and what you've been reporting, I'd like to schedule you for cataract surgery. At this time, I think we'd just do the one side.

☐ 喫煙者であったり高血圧症であったりすると、白内障の発症のリスクがより大きくなります。

The facts that you're a smoker and that you have high blood pressure put you at greater risk for developing cataracts.

☐ あなたの濁っている水晶体を取り除き、角膜の端にごく小さな切れ込みを入れて、人工の水晶体と取り替えます。

Well, we remove your lens that is cloudy and we replace it with an artificial lens, all through a tiny incision at the edge of your cornea.

▶ incision：切開、切れ込み　　cornea：角膜

☐ 多くの患者さんには、標準的な単焦点のIOL（眼内レンズ）で十分です。

For many patients, a standard single-focus IOL is just fine.

▶ IOL (Intraocular lens)：人工水晶体、眼内レンズ
＊白内障手術で曇った水晶体を摘出して、代わりに装着される人工の水晶体。

☐ 常に遠近の両方に焦点を合わせるよう設計された「多焦点」で「融通の効く」眼内レンズもあります。あなたの場合には、多焦点のレンズのものを装着することができるかもしれません。

There are also "multifocal" and "accommodating" IOLs designed to provide both distance and near close-up focus at all times. In your case, we may be able to implant one of these multifocal lenses.

▶ multifocal：多焦点の

# Chapter 22 - 耳鼻咽喉科

1 めまい・耳鳴り ●●● Dizziness

耳鼻咽喉科の Dr. Amano の診察室を訪ねている患者は、めまいの症状を訴えています。横になっても立っていても目が回るようです。

Dr. Please describe the episodes of dizziness for me.

Pt. It happens when I lie down. My eyes start moving around and I feel like something is pressing me down to the bed.

Dr. Have you noticed any other symptoms that you think might be related?

Pt. I'm not sure this has anything to do with it, but even after I get off a train, I feel like I'm still on it and my body is moving and the ground underneath me seems like it's bouncing up and down. Also, sometimes when I'm standing still, I feel like the floor is moving.

Dr. This sounds like BPPV, Benign Paroxysmal Positional Vertigo. I'd like to confirm this. We'll start with rotary-chair testing. Let's have you sit in that seat over there, which is controlled by a computer. The movement of the chair will stimulate certain reactions that we can gauge by your eye movement. This should tell us a little more.

Pt. I'm really, really dizzy now!

Dr. Yes, I can see it on the monitor. I'm going to do an adjustment now. This should give you some relief. (moves the patient's neck) Then I'm going to give you a week's worth of oral medication. For the next week or so, try to avoid looking down as much as possible. Try to hold your head straight. I'd like you to come back in when the medicine runs out. We'll reassess when I see you then.

語句・表現

BPPV (benign paroxysmal positional vertigo)：良性発作性頭位めまい

rotary-chair testing：回転椅子検査
gauge：〜を判断する、評価する

1 めまい・耳鳴り ・・・ Dizziness

訳

D：めまいの症状が起きた時のことについて説明してください。

P：横になると起こります。目が回り始め、何かが私をベッドに押し付けているかのように感じます。

D：関連があると思うような他の症状には気付かれましたか。

P：これが何か関連しているかどうかはよくわかりませんが、電車を降りても、まだ乗っているような気がして、体が動き、足元の地面が上下に跳ねるように感じます。それから、じっと立っていると、床が動いているように感じる時があります。

D：これはBPPV（良性発作性頭位めまい）のようです。これを確認したいと思います。回転椅子検査を始めます。あそこにあるコンピュータ制御の椅子に座りましょう。椅子の動きはある種の反応を引き起こし、それはあなたの目の動きによって測定できます。この検査でもう少し詳しいことがわかるはずです。

P：今、本当にすごく目が回っています。

D：はい、その様子がモニターで見えます。今ここで、（首と頭の）位置の調整を行います。これでいくらか楽になるに違いありません。（患者の首を操作する）それから、1週間分の経口薬を出します。来週あたりまで、できるだけ（立ったまま）下を見るのを避けてください。頭をまっすぐに保つようにしてください。薬がなくなった頃に診察を受けにいらしてください。次に診察に来られるときに改めて拝見しましょう。

雑学

めまい（Dizziness）

「良性発作性頭位めまい症（BPPV）」は、耳石がはがれおちることで起こります。めまいの原因はさまざまで、対処法もさまざまですが、初期症状に効くいくつかの簡単な家庭療法（home remedies）を紹介します。
① 水分補給：脱水 dehydration はめまいの原因となります。少し砂糖を加えたレモン水なら、グルコースレベルが急速に改善されるのでより有効です。
② ショウガ：めまいや車酔い効果があります。生のショウガを絞って紅茶に入れると飲みやすいです。血行が悪いことはめまいの原因のひとつですが、ショウガは血の循環を改善します。
③ セロリ：めまいの原因が貧血からきている場合には、セロリジュースがお勧めです。
④ ヨーグルト：新鮮なフルーツを入れたヨーグルトを習慣づければ、便秘も防げます。

Chapter 22 耳鼻咽喉科

耳鼻咽喉科　使える表現

症状をたずねる

☐ **Dr.** めまいについて説明していただけますか。
Could you describe the dizziness?
Pt. 部屋中を飛んでいるような感じです。／部屋が回っているような感じです。
I feel like I'm flying around the room. / It feels like the room is spinning.

☐ **Dr.** めまいの症状が起きた時のことについて説明してください。
❁ Please describe the episodes of dizziness for me.
Pt. ひどいめまいがして、常に耳鳴りがしています。
I'm very dizzy and my ears are always ringing.

☐ 関連があると思うような他の症状には気付かれましたか。
❁ Have you noticed any other symptoms that you think might be related?

☐ **Dr.** 今までにこうした症状を何か経験したことはありますか。
Have you ever had anything like this before?
Pt. いいえ、10日程前に始まったばかりです。
No, it just started about ten days ago.

☐ **Dr.** この症状はどのくらい続いていますか。
How long has this been going on? / How long does an episode last?
Pt. 時には30分あるいはそれ以上めまいや耳鳴りがします。
Sometimes I'm dizzy and my ears are ringing for half an hour or more.

診断・治療

☐ 関節炎の問題とそれに引き続いて起こる首の痛みが、めまいを引き起こすのだと思います。
I think that the arthritis problem and the subsequent pain in your neck is what's causing the dizziness.
▶ arthritis：関節炎

1 めまい・耳鳴り ... **Dizziness**

☐ 首の炎症を鎮める薬を処方します。薬でめまいと痛みは治まると思います。

I'm prescribing some medicine that should reduce the inflammation in your neck. I think this will give you less dizziness and less pain.

☐ 感染がひどい場合、鼻の後ろから中耳へと空気を送る耳管の機能が悪くなることがあります。

Sometimes when there's a lot of infection, the Eustachian tube, which carries the air from the back of your nose to your middle ear, doesn't work very well.

▶ Eustachian tube：エウスタキオ管、耳管

☐ **Pt.** コレステリン腫と診断されています。どうすればよいでしょうか。

I've been diagnosed with a cholesteatoma. What can be done for it?

Dr. 幸いさほど進行していません。まずより容易な方法で対応できると思います。

Fortunately, it hasn't progressed too far. I think we can go the easier route first.

▶ cholesteatoma：コレステリン腫

☐ 患部を十分によく洗浄してから、抗生物質と点耳剤を使って、感染を和らげられるかどうか見ましょう。

We'll clean it really well and then use antibiotics and eardrops to see if we can ease the infection.

☐ めまいが再発した場合、「エプリー法」という治療法があります。理学療法士が指導します。

If the dizziness returns, there's a technique called the "Epley Maneuver." A physical therapist can teach it to you.

☐ **Pt.** BPPV（良性発作性頭位めまい）の原因は何なのでしょうか。

Do you know what causes BPPV?

Dr. 原因はいろいろあります。加齢によって起こることもあります。あなたの耳の中の結晶がずれています。それを定位置に戻すよう調整します。

There are a variety of causes. It sometimes happens with age. There are crystals in your ears that get out of position. We're going to do an adjustment to move them back in place.

Chapter 22 - 耳鼻咽喉科

2 メニエール病 ●●● Meniere's Disease

今日、Dr. Amano の診察室を訪れている患者には、目まい、難聴、それに耳の中に圧迫感などの症状があります。

CD2-44

Dr. Could you tell me exactly what your symptoms are?

Pt. Well, I feel like I'm having some trouble hearing. Some days are worse than others.

Dr. Okay, it also says here that you feel dizzy?

Pt. Yes. That's the worst thing. I feel like I'm flying, even though I'm sitting still. I also have some ringing in my ears …

Dr. So, some hearing loss, tinnitus, that is to say, ringing in your ears, … Tell me something, do you ever feel any pressure in your ears?

Pt. Yes. I feel like my ears are full all the time.

Dr. Do you feel depressed due to the symptoms?

Pt. I'd have to say yes to that, too.

Dr. Out of curiosity, did you have any head injuries as a child?

Pt. Yes, I had to have a few stitches in my head after a fall.

Dr. Well, I believe you have Meniere's disease. We don't know all the causes, but I've had several Meniere's patients that experienced head trauma as a child.

Pt. What kind of treatment will I need? Is there a cure?

Dr. We don't exactly have a cure, but there are various drugs and strategies we can use. We'll probably start with something that will calm you down and control the vertigo. I'd like to test the dizziness with VNG, videonystagmography. This test will tell me about your balance function through your eye movement.

2 メニエール病 ●●● Meniere's Disease

訳

D： どんな症状なのかを具体的に教えていただけますか。

P： ええと、何か聞こえにくいように思います。日によってはひどいことがあります。

D： なるほど、ここにめまいがするとも書かれていますね。

P： はい。それが最悪なのです。じっと座っている時でさえ、飛んでいるように感じます。耳鳴りがすることもあります。

D： それで、難聴、耳鳴り、つまり耳の中で鳴っている感覚ですね…ちょっと教えてください、あなたは耳に何か圧力を感じたりしますか。

P： はい。いつでも耳の中がいっぱいになっているように感じます。

D： その症状のために気が滅入ったりしますか。

P： そのことについてもはいと答えざるを得ません。

D： 参考までに、あなたは子供のときに頭にけがをしたことがありましたか。

P： はい、落下して、頭を数針縫わなければなりませんでした。

D： ええと、あなたはメニエール病でしょう。すべての原因を把握しているわけではありませんが、幼少期に頭に外傷を受けた経験を持つメニエール病の患者さんを何人か診たことがあります。

P： 私にはどんな類の治療が必要なのでしょうか。治療法はありますか。

D： 確実な治療法はありませんが、私たちが活用できる薬や対処法はたくさんあります。あなたを落ち着かせてめまいをコントロールするようなものから始めることになるでしょう。VNG（ビデオ式眼振計測装置）を使っためまいの検査をしたいと思います。この検査は、あなたの目の動きを通してバランス機能を測るものです。

語句・表現

hearing loss：難聴、聴力損失［低下］
tinnitus：耳鳴り

VNG, videonystagmography：VNG（ビデオ式眼振計測装置）、VNG検査

Chapter 22 耳鼻咽喉科

●●● 耳鼻咽喉科　使える表現

症状をたずねる

☐ **Dr.** あなたは耳に何か圧力を感じたりしますか。
　✿ Do you ever feel any pressure in your ears?
　Pt. はい。いつでも耳の中がいっぱいになっているように感じます。
　✿ Yes. I feel like my ears are full all the time.

☐ **Dr.** あなたの病歴には何も書かれていないようですが、ひょっとして、子供のときに頭にけがをなさいましたか。

　　I don't see anything in your medical history, but did you, by any chance, have a head injury as a child?
　Pt. はい、私は兄と熊手で落ち葉を掃いていて、兄がうっかり熊手で私の頭を打ちました。
　　Yes, I was raking leaves with my brother and he accidentally hit me in the head with his rake.
　　　▶ rake leaves：落ち葉を掃く

診断・処方

☐ あなたから伺ったことと、VNG評価から見て、あなたはメニエール病にかかっていると思います。

　Based on what you've told me and the results of the VNG evaluation, I believe that you're suffering from Meniere's disease.

☐ あなたはメニエール病だと思います。内耳にある液体の組成あるいは量に問題が生じているのが原因のようです。

　I believe you have Meniere's disease. It seems to be caused by a problem with the composition or volume of the fluid in the inner ear.

☐ すべての原因を把握しているわけではありませんが、幼少期に頭に外傷を受けた経験を持つメニエール病の患者さんを何人か診たことがあります。
　✿ We don't know all the causes, but I've had several Meniere's patients that experienced head trauma as a child.

2 メニエール病 ●●● Meniere's Disease

☐ **Dr.** 簡単で即効性のある治療法がメニエール病にない理由の一つは、この病気にはさまざまな要因が関わっていることだと思います。

We think that one of the reasons that there is no easy and fast cure for Meniere's disease is that there are a variety of factors involved.

Pt. では、私はどうするべきでしょうか。

So what should I do?

Dr. 私たちが話し合った治療方法を守り、落ち込まないように心がけてください。多くの人たちが、症状が緩和され、めまいの発作が治まっています。

Stick to the treatment plan we've discussed and try not to get depressed. Many people go into remission and stop having the dizzy spells.

▶ go into remission：（症状などが）緩和される　　dizzy spell：めまいの発作

☐ まず、軽度の精神安定剤を処方しようと思いますが、それでめまいの発作が今より我慢できるようにもなるでしょう。

I think the first thing to do is to use a mild tranquilizer, which will also make the dizzy spells more tolerable.

▶ tranquilizer：精神安定剤、鎮痛剤

☐ 即効性のある薬ですから、とりあえず、精神安定剤から始めましょう。うまくいけば、栄養補給剤へ切り替えられると思います。

Let's start with the tranquilizer for now, because it's fast-acting. Hopefully, we can transition you to some supplements.

▶ fast-acting：即効性のある

雑学
メニエール病（Meniere's disease）

　フランスの医師プロスペル・メニエール（Prosper Ménière）が1861年に初めてめまいの原因の一つに内耳性のものがあることを報告したことからこの名前がついています。「メニエル病」「メヌエル病」「メニエール氏病」とも言われます。

　メニエール病患者でありながら月に降り立った宇宙飛行士がいるのをご存知でしょうか。アメリカの宇宙飛行士アラン・シェパードです。めまいの発作を繰り返しながらもその後も月への情熱を失わず、発症から5年後、内リンパ嚢手術を受けたシェパードは、めまい発作から完全に解放されました。シェパードは、アポロ14号の船長として月面に降り立ったのです。

3 鼻炎・副鼻腔炎 ●●● Rhinitis/Sinus Infections

Dr. Amano を訪れた患者は鼻水やくしゃみを訴えています。典型的なアレルギー性鼻炎の症状のようです。

Dr. My preliminary assessment is that you have allergic rhinitis.

Pt. I doubt I'm allergic to rhinoceroses, so you must be referring to inflammation of the nose. Luckily, I studied a little Greek through word etymology. We never use the word "rhinitis" in conversation in the States.

Dr. As a physician and an allergy researcher, it's interesting to me that although they may not have heard the term rhinitis, Americans often talk to me about their sinuses. In Japan, everyone knows rhinitis, but they don't seem to have an awareness of sinuses and sinusitis.

Pt. I think we hear a lot about sinus pain in TV commercials.

Dr. Right. I worked in the U.S. for a year when I was younger. So perhaps if I were an American doctor, I'd be telling you that I think you have classic nasal allergies. Based on your symptoms, I don't think your sinuses are involved. You appear to have nasal congestion and a runny nose with clear mucus. You also report frequent sneezing and complain of itchiness in your ears. These are all symptoms of allergic rhinitis.

Pt. What do I need to do?

Dr. I'll prescribe some allergy medication, but first I want to run a few tests.

Pt. OK. Got it.

語句・表現

allergic rhinitis：アレルギー性鼻炎
etymology：語源
sinus：洞、副鼻腔（複数形：sinuses）
sinusitis：副鼻腔炎
nasal congestion：鼻づまり
mucus：粘液

3 鼻炎・副鼻腔炎　Rhinitis / Sinus Infections

訳

D：初見では、あなたはアレルギー性鼻炎です。

P：私がrhinoceroses（サイ）に対してアレルギーがあるとは思えないので、先生は鼻の炎症のことをおっしゃっているに違いありません。幸い、私はギリシア語を、語源を通して少々勉強しました（だから理解できたのですが）。米国では、私たちが会話の中でrhinitis（鼻炎）という単語を使うことはありません。

D：医師でアレルギー研究者である私にとって、これは興味深いことです。つまり、アメリカ人はrhinitis（鼻炎）という単語は聞いたことはないかもしれませんが、よくsinuses（副鼻腔）のことを話します。日本では、鼻炎ならだれでも知っていますが、副鼻腔や副鼻腔炎のことは知らないようです。

P：テレビコマーシャルで副鼻腔の痛みについてよく聞くと思います。

D：そうですね。私は若い頃1年間米国で働いていました。ですから、もし私がアメリカ人の医師なら、「あなたは典型的な鼻アレルギーだと思います」と伝えるでしょう。症状からすると、副鼻腔は関わりがないと思うのです。あなたには、鼻づまりと、透明な粘液の鼻水の症状が出ています。頻繁なくしゃみや耳のかゆみも報告されています。これらはみな、アレルギー性鼻炎の症状です。

P：私はどうすればよいのでしょうか。

D：いくつかアレルギーの薬を処方しますが、最初に、いくつか検査を受けていただきたいと思います。

P：はい。わかりました。

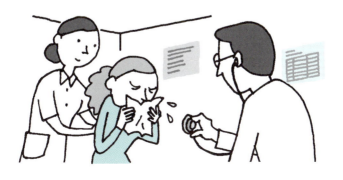

Chapter 22 - 耳鼻咽喉科

●●● 耳鼻咽喉科　使える表現

症状をたずねる

☐ よく鼻がつまりますか。
Do you often have a stuffy nose?

☐ 鼻汁はのどの方に流れていきますか。
Does the nasal mucus drain into the throat?

☐ 鼻で息をするのが苦しいですか。
Do you have difficulty breathing through your nose?

☐ 鼻にけがをしたことがありますか。
Have you had any injuries to your nose?

☐ 右側に少し鼻づまりがあるようです。
You seem a little congested on the right side.

診察

☐ 鼻の構造をチェックして、何か軟骨にゆがみがないか確認しましょう。
I want to check the structure of your nose and see if there is any deviation of the cartilage.
▶ cartilage：軟骨

☐ 片方の鼻の穴を私の親指でふさぎますので、息を吸ってみてください。
I'm going to block your nostril off with my thumb and ask you to breathe in.
▶ nostril：鼻孔（鼻の穴）

☐ 頭を私の方に上げてもらえますか。あなたの鼻を別の角度から見ることができますので。
Could you tilt your head up for me? This gives me a different view of your nose.
▶ tilt one's ～ up：～を上に傾ける

☐ 頭を上げて天井を見ていただけると、鼻を下から見られるのですが。
If you could tilt your head up and look at the ceiling, so I can see your nose from below.

3 鼻炎・副鼻腔炎　Rhinitis / Sinus Infections

☐ 横を向いてください。あなたの鼻の中心線にどこか骨が隆起しているところ、あるいはくぼんでいるところがないかを確認したいと思います。

Please turn to the side. I want to see whether or not there's a bony bump in the center of your nose, or any depressions.

▶ bony：骨ばった　　bump：隆起

☐ 鼻先から上くちびる、すなわち鼻唇までの角度を測りたいと思います。

I also want to gauge the angle from the tip of your nose to the upper lip, the nasolabial angle.

▶ nasolabial angle：鼻唇角

診断・処置

☐ 初見では、あなたはアレルギー性鼻炎です。

❂ My preliminary assessment is that you have allergic rhinitis.

☐ 鼻づまりと、透明な粘液の鼻水の症状が出ています。頻繁なくしゃみや耳のかゆみも報告されています。これらはみなアレルギー性鼻炎の症状です。

❂ You appear to have nasal congestion and a runny nose with clear mucus. You also report frequent sneezing and complain of itchiness in your ears. These are all symptoms of allergic rhinitis.

☐ 私が行った検査によると、あなたが鼻中隔彎曲症であるのは明らかです。

Based on my examination, it's clear that you have a deviated septum.

▶ deviated septum (DNS)：鼻中隔彎曲（症）

☐ 鼻のステロイド・スプレーの処方を始めたいと思います。この症状に飲み薬なしで対処できるか様子を見ましょう。

I'd like to start you out on a nasal steroid spray. Let's see if we can deal with this without oral medication.

☐ もう一つの選択肢は、矯正手術です。

The other alternative is corrective surgery.

▶ corrective surgery：矯正手術

4 耳感染症 ●●● Ear Infections

Chapter 22 - 耳鼻咽喉科

今日、Dr. Amano の診察室を訪れた患者は、このところ右の耳にトラブルを抱えています。耳垂れも始まったようです。

Dr. Could you explain what's going on with your ear? You said the problem was with the right one?

Pt. Yes. I've had a pain in my ear for the last week. I'm even having a little trouble hearing.

Dr. Have you had any fluid draining from this ear?

Pt. Yes. I had that yesterday. That's the reason I decided to come in today.

Dr. How about allergies?

Pt. Yes. I had a flare-up with my allergy to Japanese cedar a couple of weeks ago.

Dr. When you have a cold, the flu, or allergies, there is the possibility of an ear infection. This might hurt a bit, but I'd like to take a quick look in both ears. Okay, there will be a little puff of air. … Ah yes, this is normal. Now let me look at the right one…

Pt. It's bad?

Dr. Well, it's definitely filled with fluid. The puff of air causes the eardrum to move in a healthy ear, which it did when I used the pneumatic otoscope on your left ear, but the right one didn't move, which means it's filled with fluid. This is why your hearing is not as good as usual.

Pt. What should I do?

Dr. I recommend you use a warm compress on your ear. I'm also going to prescribe some eardrops. Is the pain so bad that you think you need pain medication?

Pt. No. I can handle it.

4 耳感染症 ●●● Ear Infections

訳

D：耳の状態について説明していただけますか。右の耳に問題があるとのことですね。

P：はい。ここ1週間、耳が痛みます。少し聞こえにくいことすらあります。

D：こちらの耳からの耳垂れはありますか。

P：はい。昨日ありました。今日、診察に来たのはそのためです。

D：アレルギーはありますか。

P：はい。数週間前、私は杉に対するアレルギーを急に再発しました。

D：風邪やインフルエンザだったり、アレルギーを発症していたりすると、耳の感染症になる可能性があります。少し痛いかもしれませんが、両耳を素早くチェックしたいと思います。結構です。少し空気を入れますよ。ああ、こちらは正常です。では、右耳を見せてください。

P：悪いのでしょうか。

D：そうですね、液体で満たされています。健康な耳では、空気を吹き込むと鼓膜が動きます。気密耳鏡を使った検査で、このことを左耳で確認しましたが、右耳では動きませんでした。つまり右耳には液体が溜まっているということです。このためにあなたはいつもより聞こえにくいのです。

P：どうすればいいでしょうか。

D：耳に温湿布をするようお勧めします。点耳剤も処方しましょう。鎮痛剤が必要だと感じるほど痛みはひどいでしょうか。

P：いいえ。自分で対処できます。

語句・表現

flare-up：急激な再発
puff：（空気や煙などが）一吹きすること
eardrum：鼓膜
pneumatic otoscope：気密耳鏡　＊外耳道圧を変化させて鼓膜の可動性を観察する器具。
eardrops：点耳剤
pain medication：鎮痛剤

耳鼻咽喉科　使える表現

症状をたずねる

☐ 耳の状態について説明していただけますか。右の耳に問題があるとのことですね。

❀ Could you explain what's going on with your ear? You said the problem was with the right one?

☐ 耳の調子がよくないのですか。

Are your ears bothering you?

☐ こちらの耳からの耳垂れはありますか。

❀ Have you had any fluid draining from this ear?

☐ 熱を下げるのに、市販の薬を飲んでいますか。

Have you been taking any over-the-counter medication to reduce the fever?

☐ 鎮痛剤が必要だと感じるほど痛みはひどいでしょうか。

❀ Is the pain so bad that you think you need pain medication?

☐ **Dr.** 小児科の伊藤先生が、お子さんの耳をもっとよく診てもらうようにとのことで、こちらへ来られたのですね。彼女は話せますか。

I see that Dr. Ito from our pediatrics department sent you over to see if I can get a better look at her ear. Does she speak?

Pt. ほんの2、3言です。まだ14ヶ月で、耳の調子が悪くなって以来、不機嫌なのです。

Just a few words. She's only 14 months and she's been in a bad mood since the trouble with her ear started.

診断

☐ この症状は、典型的な中耳炎という感染症のようです。

This looks like typical otitis media, a middle ear infection.
　　▶ otitis media：中耳炎

☐ ちょっと見せてください。確かに耳の感染症ですね。

Let's take a look. You definitely have an ear infection.

4 耳感染症 ●●● Ear Infections

☐ otitis mediaは、耳の感染症を表す医学用語です。つまり、中耳の炎症のことです。

Otitis media is just a fancy medical term for an ear infection— an infection of the middle ear, actually.

☐ 風邪やインフルエンザだったり、アレルギーを発症していると、耳の感染症になる可能性があります。

✿▶When you have a cold, the flu, or allergies, there's the possibility of an ear infection.

☐ 大人よりも子供たちの方が耳の感染症にかかりやすいのです。実際に、子供たちの75％が3歳になるまでに耳の感染症になっています。

Children experience many more ear infections than adults. Actually, 75% of children will have an ear infection by age three.

☐ 子供たちは、耳管が短くて平らなので、私たちのような大人よりも耳の形状がまっすぐです。そのために黴菌が侵入しやすいのです。

Children have shorter and more horizontal Eustachian tubes that are straighter than ours. This makes it easy for bacteria to get in.

▶ Eustachian tube：耳管

処置・処方

☐ この耳の感染症の治療のため、これからの2週間、抗生物質を服用していただきます。

I'm going to want you to take antibiotics for the next two weeks to get rid of this ear infection.

☐ 耳に温湿布をするようお勧めします。点耳剤も処方しましょう。

✿▶I recommend you use a warm compress on your ear. I'm also going to prescribe some eardrops.

☐ お子さんに点耳剤使うとき、外耳道に直接入れないようにしてください、痛みますので。

When you apply your child's eardrops, please do not drop them directly into the ear canal, this could be painful.

Chapter 23 歯科・口腔外科

1　歯根管　●●● Root Canals

歯科・口腔外科医の Dr. Okuma は神経の痛みを訴える患者に歯根管の手術を勧めます。このところ痛みが引いているので手術には抵抗があるようです。

Dr. You say you've been experiencing pain when you chew?

Pt. Yes. It's felt like something was wrong for a few weeks. I was getting pain all the way up my jaw. I thought it might be nerve pain.

Dr. Do you have any sensitivity to hot or cold foods?

Pt. Yes.

Dr. Does it go away right away or does it linger?

Pt. I'd say it lingers.

Dr. I'm going to take a look. Open wide … (pause) All right, you'll need to make an appointment with one of our oral surgeon for root canal surgery.

Pt. The pain has actually not been as bad as it was for the last few days.

Dr. That's because the nerve is starting to die. The oral surgeon will drill right through the crown you have, clean it out completely and shape the root canal, then, fill it with a biocompatible material and seal it with temporary materials. You'll come back to me afterward, and I'll put in a new filling. Once the tooth has been refilled and heals, you should be pain free.

Pt. I was told that in Japan dentists do surgery themselves.

Dr. It depends on the dental practice. At this hospital, we specialize in different, specific areas, so the oral surgeons are able to use state-of-the-art microsurgery tools. This use of specialists might be similar to what you had back home.

Pt. Yes, where I'm from, we have to go to an oral surgeon even for an extraction.

1 歯根管 ●●● Root Canals

訳

D：噛むときに痛みがあるとのことですね。

P：はい。ここ数週間、どこか悪いように感じています。あごまで痛みが広がりました。神経の痛みのように思いました。

D：熱いものや冷たいものが歯にしみますか。

P：はい。

D：その痛みはすぐに消えますか、それともいつまでも残りますか。

P：いつまでも残るように思います。

D：拝見しましょう。口を大きく開けてください。(中断) はい、結構です。あなたは、歯根管の手術のため、当院の口腔外科医の予約を入れる必要があります。

P：実を言うと、痛みはここ数日間あまりひどくありませんが。

D：それは神経が死に始めているからです。口腔外科医は、症状のある歯冠に穴を空け、感染をすっかり除去し、歯根管を成形してから、生体適合性のある材料を詰め、仮の材料をかぶせます。後日、再診されたときに、新しい詰め物を装填します。いったん詰め物を入れ替えて治癒すれば、痛みから解放されるはずです。

P：日本の歯医者さんは手術も自分たちで行うと伺いましたが。

D：歯科診療の仕方次第です。当院では、私たちは幅広い専門分野に精通していますので、口腔外科医は最新のマイクロサージェリー技法を使うことができます。こうした専門医による治療法は、あなたが本国で受けてきたものと似ているかもしれません。

P：はい、私の国では、抜歯ですら口腔外科医を訪ねなければなりません。

語句・表現

linger：いつまでも残る
oral surgeon：口腔外科医
biocompatible：生体適合性のある

Chapter 23 歯科・口腔外科

●●● 歯科・口腔外科　使える表現

症状をたずねる

☐ 歯茎が痛みますか。
Do you have pain in your gums?

☐ ぐらぐらする歯がありますか。
Do any of your teeth feel loose?

☐ 歯茎がどこか腫れていますか。
Are the gums around any of your teeth swollen?

☐ 歯を磨くと歯茎から出血しますか。
Do your gums bleed when you brush your teeth?

☐ 噛むときに痛みがあるとのことですね。
❀ You say you've been experiencing pain when you chew?

☐ 熱い物や冷たい物が歯にしみますか。
❀ Do you have any sensitivity to hot or cold foods?

☐ その痛みはすぐに消えますか、それともいつまでも残りますか
❀ Does it go away right away or does it linger?

診察

☐ その症状は歯根の表面の一部が露出し、ごくわずかに歯茎が後退することによって起こった可能性があります。
I think it may be caused by very slight gum recession that is exposing a small part of the root surface.

☐ あなたには明らかに膿瘍がありますね。これは歯茎の膿瘍でしょう。
You clearly have an abscess ... I think this is a gum abscess.
▶ abscess：膿瘍（膿がたまった状態）

☐ 感染があごや首にまで進んできているようです。しこりが感じ取れますか。
I can see the infection has worked its way down your jaw and neck. Feel this lump?

1 歯根管　Root Canals

☐ これは膿瘍によるものです。今、膿を出してこれを治療しますから、我慢してください

This is from the abscess. I'm going to drain the pus and treat it now.

☐ それは神経が死に始めているからです。

➤ That's because the nerve is starting to die.

☐ そのままにしておくと腐ってしまいます。

If we leave it in, it will start to rot.

☐ これは感染しているように思います。レントゲン写真を撮り、感染がどのくらいまで広がっているかを確認したいと思います。

I think this might be an infection. I want to take some X-rays to see how far the infection has spread.

☐ これによって手術が必要となる場合に、歯根管がどのくらいの長さであるかもわかります。

This will also show us how long the root canals of your teeth are, and if you require surgery.

治療・助言

☐ 抗生物質と鎮痛剤を処方します。

I am going to prescribe a course of antibiotics and pain killers.

☐ 後日、再診されたときに、新しい詰め物を装填します。

➤ You'll come back to me afterward, and I will put in a new filling.

☐ 横向きに歯を磨くと露出した歯根の表面を摩耗させますから、必ず歯を上下に磨くようにしてください。

I want you to be sure to brush up and down, as brushing sideways wears away exposed root surfaces.

☐ 将来的には、上あごの歯をある時点で抜くか、下あごの歯の位置にインプラントを埋め込むことを考える必要があるでしょう。

We will either have to extract the top tooth at some point in the future, or consider putting an implant where the bottom tooth was.

雑学

Lay terms（一般用語）とProfessional terms（専門用語）

　医療に関わる人たちがお互いに用いる言葉は専門的で患者さんにはわかりにくいものです。2通りの用語は、PART 1（基礎編）P.47でもいくつか紹介しましたが、ここでもさらに、よく用いられる用語を紹介しましょう。

Lay term(s)		Professional term(s)
bruise	あざ、打撲傷	contusion
mumps	おたふくかぜ	epidemic parotitis
thumb	親指	pollex
itching	かゆみ	pruritus
lump	こぶ	mass
pinkie; pinky, little finger	小指	digitus minimus
piles	痔	hemorrhoids
frozen shoulder	四十肩	adhesive capsulitis

＊日本語のように40-year-old shoulderと言うこともあります。

hives	じんましん	urticaria
shingles	帯状疱疹	herpes zoster virus
morning sickness	つわり	hyperemesis gravidarum
middle finger	中指	digitus medius
pimples	にきび	acne (vulgaris)
nauseous	吐き気を催す	nauseated
measles	はしか	rubeola; morbilli

＊read measlesやfive-day measlesと言うこともあります。

snot	鼻水	mucus
trigger finger	ばね指	stenosing tenosynovitis

＊イギリス英語では日本語のようにspring fingerと言うこともあります。

index finger	人差し指	digitus secundus manus
ring finger	薬指	digitus annularis
German measles	三日ばしか	rubella

＊日本語のようにthree-day measlesと言うこともあります。

swollen glands	リンパの腫れ	adenopathy; lymphadenopathy

医療用語リスト

本文中で紹介した医療用語の中から重要度の高いものを、アルファベット順にリストにしてあります。本文ページ数も示してありますので、英文索引としてもご利用ください。

A		
☐ abscess	膿瘍（膿がたまった状態）	288
☐ acetaminophen	アセトアミノフェン	206
☐ acid reflux	胃酸の逆流	131
☐ acid-blocking medication	制酸剤	110
☐ acute pain	急性の痛み	39
☐ allergic rhinitis	アレルギー性鼻炎	278
☐ alopecia areata	円形脱毛症	260
☐ alzheimer's disease	アルツハイマー病	214
☐ anesthesia	麻酔	86
☐ anesthesiologist	麻酔医	87
☐ anesthetic	麻酔薬	86, 101
☐ aneurism	動脈瘤	213
☐ angina	狭心症	131
☐ anoscope	肛門鏡、直腸鏡	226
☐ anoscopy	肛門鏡検査（法）	228
☐ antibiotics	抗生剤	149, 177
☐ antidepressant	抗うつ剤	165
☐ antihistamin	抗ヒスタミン剤	250
☐ anti-inflammatory effect	抗炎症作用	101
☐ anus	肛門	238
☐ appendectomy	虫垂切除術	174
☐ appendicitis	虫垂炎	174
☐ arrhythmia	不整脈	135
☐ arteriosclerosis	動脈硬化	140
☐ arthritis	関節炎	272
☐ asthma	ぜんそく	222
☐ atrial flutter	心房粗動（不整脈の一種）	132
☐ attack	発作	106
☐ autoimmune disease	自己免疫疾患（AID）	148
☐ autoimmune disorders	自己免疫疾患（AID）	258

B		
☐ backache	腰痛、背痛	35, 182
☐ benign	良性の	230
☐ beta blocker	ベータブロッカー	128, 143
☐ bile	胆汁	110
☐ biocompatible	生体適合性のある	286
☐ biologic	生物製剤	173
☐ biopsy	バイオプシー、生体組織検査	146

☐	bipolar disorder	双極性障害	166
☐	black eye	（目のまわりの）青あざ、黒あざ	188
☐	bladder	膀胱	238
☐	bladder stone	膀胱結石	242
☐	blepharitis	眼瞼炎	265
☐	blink	まばたきをする	246
☐	bloated	むくんだ	114
☐	blood donation	輸血	86
☐	blood test	血液検査	69, 115
☐	BMD	骨塩定量測定検査	69
☐	bone density test	骨密度検査	64, 69
☐	BPPV	良性発作性頭位めまい	270
☐	brain trauma	脳損傷	213
☐	breast growths	乳腺腫瘍	218
☐	breast surgery	乳腺外科	12
☐	bronchoscopy	気管支鏡検査	69
☐	bruit	雑音	140

C

☐	caesarean section	帝王切開	236
☐	cancerous	がんの、がん性の	230
☐	carbohydrates	炭水化物	154, 160
☐	cardiac catheterization	心臓カテーテル法	143
☐	cardiovascular medicine	循環器内科	12
☐	cardiovascular surgery	心臓血管外科	12
☐	cardioversion	電気的除細動	132
☐	carpal tunnel syndrome	手根管症候群	196
☐	cataracts	白内障	266
☐	catheterization	カテーテル法	205
☐	CBC	完全血球算定	149, 150
☐	chemotherapy	化学療法	245
☐	chest pains	胸の痛み	35
☐	childbirth	分娩	234
☐	chronic coughing	慢性咳嗽（がいそう）	194
☐	chronic pain	慢性痛、慢性の痛み	98
☐	click-murmur syndrome	クリック音症候群	128
☐	clonic seizure	間代発作	209
☐	colonoscopy	大腸内視鏡検査	69, 108
☐	coma	昏睡	213
☐	combination therapy	併用療法	257

☐	compress	湿布	105
☐	compulsion	衝動脅迫	161
☐	consent form	同意書	58
☐	conservative treatment	保存療法、対処療法	263
☐	contrast dye	造影剤	241
☐	cool compresses	冷湿布	225
☐	COPD	慢性閉塞性肺疾患	118
☐	cornea	角膜	269
☐	cortisone	コーチゾン	101
☐	cough	咳	33
☐	CPAP machine	CPAP装置	126
☐	CPR	心肺機能蘇	92
☐	crutch	松葉杖	186
☐	CSF (cerebrospinal fluid)	脳脊髄液	102
☐	CT Scan	CTスキャン	69
☐	cyst	嚢腫(のうしゅ)	218
☐	cystitis	膀胱炎	238
☐	cystoscopy	膀胱鏡検査	69, 241

D

☐	dehydrated	脱水状態の	217, 225
☐	dehydration	脱水	214
☐	dementia	認知症	216
☐	dentistry and oral surgery	歯科・口腔外科	12
☐	depressed	うつ状態の	163
☐	depression	うつ病	162
☐	dermatology	皮膚科	12
☐	deviated septum (DNS)	鼻中隔彎曲(症)	281
☐	diabetes	糖尿病	154
☐	dialysis	透析	116
☐	diarrhea	下痢	33, 106
☐	digital exam (examination)	指診	226
☐	discharge	分泌	232
☐	disk herniation	椎間板ヘルニア	196
☐	dissolvable stitch	溶ける縫合糸	193
☐	diuretic	利尿剤	117
☐	dizziiness	めまい	270
☐	dominant hand	利き手	196
☐	drip	点滴	225
☐	drool	よだれを垂らす	246

☐	drops	点眼薬	263
☐	dry eye syndrome	ドライアイ	262
☐	dry patch	ドライスポット	263
☐	dull pain	鈍い痛み	39

E

☐	ear infections	耳感染症	282
☐	earache	耳痛	35
☐	eardrops	点耳剤	282
☐	eardrum	鼓膜	282
☐	eating disorders	摂食障害	158
☐	EEG (Electroencephalogram)	脳波検査	69
☐	EKG [ECG]	心電図	64, 69
☐	embolization	塞栓術	230
☐	Emergency Room: ER	救急外来	12
☐	emphysema	肺気腫	121
☐	endocrinology and metabolism	糖尿病代謝内科	12
☐	endoscopic exam [test]	内視鏡検査	64
☐	endoscopy	内視鏡検査	69
☐	enlarged prostate	前立腺肥大	242
☐	ENT (ear nose throat)	耳鼻咽喉科	102
☐	entail	〜を引き起こす、伴う	143
☐	epilepsy	てんかん	206
☐	eustachian tube	エウスタキオ管、耳管	273
☐	exhalation	呼気	123
☐	exhale	息を吐く	123
☐	eye test	眼の検査	69

F

☐	facial droop	顔面下垂	246
☐	facial paralysis	顔面神経痛	246
☐	faint	気絶する、失神する	132
☐	fast arrhythmia	徐脈性不整脈	135
☐	fast-acting	即効性のある	277
☐	fever	熱	33
☐	fibroid	子宮筋腫	230
☐	first visit	初診	14, 20
☐	flare-up	急激な再発	282
☐	flu	インフルエンザ	222
☐	flu shot	インフルエンザの予防注射	42

☐	foul mood	不機嫌、憂うつ	167
☐	fractures	骨折	186
☐	frown	眉をひそめる、顔をしかめる	246
☐	fundal height	子宮底長	236

G

☐	gallbladder	胆嚢（のう）	179
☐	gallstones	胆石	178
☐	gastroenterology	消化器内科	12
☐	gastroscopy	胃内視鏡検査	69
☐	GCS	グラスゴー・コーマ・スケール	92
☐	general anesthesia	全身麻酔	87, 229
☐	general surgery	一般外科	12
☐	GFR	糸球体ろ過率	114
☐	GI series	消化器造影	66, 69
☐	Gleason score	グリソンスコア（がんの悪性度を示す）	245
☐	glucose level	血糖値	154
☐	glycemic index (GI)	グリセミック指数、血糖指数	154
☐	glycemic load (GL)	血糖負荷	154
☐	groin	鼠径（そけい）部	194

H

☐	hair loss	抜け毛	258
☐	hardening	硬化	140
☐	hay fever	花粉症	210
☐	headache	頭痛	35, 102
☐	health examinations	健康診断	13
☐	health insurance card	健康保険証	21
☐	heart rate	心拍数	132
☐	hearing loss	難聴、聴力損失［低下］	274
☐	hearing test	聴力検査	64, 69
☐	heart disease	心臓疾患	128, 132
☐	heart rate Doppler	ドップラー心拍計	234
☐	heartburn [indigestion]	胸焼け	35, 174
☐	hematology	血液内科	12
☐	hemodialysis	血液透析	117
☐	hemoglobin A1c	ヘモグロビン・エーワンシー	154
☐	hemorrhoidectomy	痔核切除	229
☐	hemorrhoids	痔核	226
☐	hepatitis	肝臓炎、肝炎	148

☐	hernia	ヘルニア	194
☐	high blood pressure	高血圧症	136
☐	hives	じんましん	250
☐	hospital departments	診療科	12
☐	hospital ID card	診察券	22
☐	hot flash	ほてり	232
☐	humidifier	加湿器	105
☐	hypodermic needle	皮下注射針	157

I

☐	ibuprofen	イブプロフェン	110
☐	imagining tests	画像検査	115
☐	immunotherapy	免疫療法	257
☐	implantable loop recorder (ILR)	埋め込み式ループレコーダー	135
☐	incision	切開、切れ込み	179, 269
☐	infection	感染症	102
☐	inflammation	炎症	108
☐	inguinal hernia	鼠径ヘルニア	194
☐	inhalation	吸入	123
☐	Intensive Care Unit (ICU)	集中治療室	13
☐	intervention	医療介入	210, 266
☐	intravenous fluid	静脈内輸液、点滴剤	225
☐	iron deficiency	鉄欠乏	150
☐	irritant	刺激性のもの	105
☐	ischemic heart disease	虚血性心疾患	202
☐	itchy	かゆい	33

J

☐	jaundiced	黄疸にかかった	179
☐	jitteriness	神経過敏	209

K

☐	kidney biopsy	腎生検	115
☐	kidney failure [disease]	腎臓病	114

L

☐	laboratory	検査部門	13
☐	laboratory and other facilities	診察設備	13
☐	laceration	裂傷	192
☐	laparoscopically	腹腔鏡下で	174

☐	laparoscopy	腹腔鏡検査	69
☐	lesion	（皮膚の）損傷、病気	258
☐	lightheadedness	立ちくらみ	128
☐	liquid nitrogen	液体窒素	254
☐	lump	腫れ物、しこり	34, 218
☐	lumpectomy	腫瘍摘出手術	220
☐	lung function test	肺機能検査	64, 69
☐	lupus	狼瘡、ループス	258
☐	lymph node	リンパ節	146, 221
☐	lymphoma	リンパ腫	146

M

☐	malignancy	悪性腫瘍	221, 229
☐	malignant	悪性の	230, 256
☐	mammogram	マンモグラフィー、乳房X線写真	68, 218
☐	mannitol	マンニトール	117
☐	masked hypertension	仮面高血圧	137
☐	medical certificate	診断書	27
☐	medical questionnaire	問診票	20
☐	medical record	カルテ、医療記録	170
☐	meibomian glands	マイボーム腺	263
☐	Meniere's disease	メニエール病	274
☐	meningitis	髄膜炎	102
☐	menstruating	月経中の	150
☐	microsurgery	顕微鏡（下）手術	196
☐	migraine headache	偏頭痛	105
☐	mitral valve	僧帽弁	128
☐	modality	治療法	230
☐	mood	不機嫌、憂うつ	167
☐	mood swings	気分変動	168
☐	MRI	磁気共鳴映像法	69, 230
☐	mucus	粘液	118, 278
☐	muscle aches	筋肉痛	35
☐	muscle relaxant [relaxer]	筋肉弛緩剤	182
☐	MVP (mitral valve prolapse)	僧帽弁逸脱	128
☐	myocardial ischemia	心筋虚血	204

N

☐	nagging pain	しつこい痛み	39
☐	nasal congestion	鼻づまり	278

☐	nasolabial angle	鼻唇角	281
☐	nausea	吐き気	33
☐	nephrologist	腎臓専門医	114
☐	nephrology	腎臓内科	12
☐	nerve conduction	神経伝導	196
☐	nerve entrapment	神経絞扼	98
☐	nerve pain	神経痛	98
☐	neurology	神経内科	12
☐	neurosurgery	脳神経外科	12
☐	non-surgical	手術を行わない	230
☐	nostril	鼻孔（鼻の穴）	280
☐	nuclear stress test	心血管造影検査	131
☐	numb	しびれて感覚がない	39
☐	numbness	しびれ	39, 100
☐	nursing department	看護部	13

O

☐	obesity [overweight]	肥満	141
☐	obstetrics and gynecology	産婦人科	12
☐	obstructive sleep apnea	閉塞性睡眠時無呼吸	124
☐	oncologist	がん（腫瘍）専門医	233
☐	onset	発病	170
☐	operating room	手術室	13
☐	ophthalmology	眼科	12
☐	oral surgeon	口腔外科医	286
☐	orthopedic surgery	整形外科	12
☐	otorhinolaryngology	耳鼻咽喉科	12

P

☐	pain in the side	脇腹の痛み	35
☐	painkiller	鎮痛剤	98
☐	pant	荒い息をする、息を切らす	118
☐	pathology	病理、病状	256
☐	patient ID card	診察券	90
☐	pediatrics	小児科	12
☐	PEFR	最大呼気速度	122
☐	perforation	穿孔	113
☐	pericarditis	心膜炎	131
☐	pernicious anemia	悪性貧血	150
☐	pharmacy	薬剤部	13

	English	Japanese	Page
☐	phlegm	痰	118
☐	physical therapy	理学療法	213
☐	piercing pain	刺し込む痛み	39
☐	pins and needles	うずくような痛み	39
☐	plastic surgery	形成外科	12
☐	pneumatic otoscope	気密耳鏡	282
☐	postsurgical complication	術後合併症	81
☐	precaution	予防策、予防措置	98
☐	prenatal care	妊婦健診（健康診査）	234
☐	prescribe	処方する	74
☐	prescription	処方箋	73, 74, 90
☐	pressure on the nerve	神経圧迫	101
☐	proctology	肛門科	12
☐	prognosis	予後（診断）	149
☐	prostate	前立腺	242
☐	prostate biopsy	前立腺生検	245
☐	protrude	はみ出る、突き出る	228
☐	psychiatry	神経科	12
☐	pubic bone	恥骨	236
☐	pulmonary function tests	肺機能検査	122

R

	English	Japanese	Page
☐	radiation	放射線治療	220
☐	radiology	放射線	13
☐	radiology department	放射線科	242
☐	rash	湿疹	34, 250
☐	reaction	反応、副作用	98
☐	reassess	〜を再評価する、見直す	110
☐	rebound tenderness	反跳痛	174
☐	rectal exam	直腸検査	242
☐	regimen	投薬・治療計画	253, 265
☐	registration form	診療申込書	20
☐	rehabilitation	リハビリテーション	13
☐	renal failure	腎不全	116
☐	reproductive plan	出産計画	233
☐	respiratory medicine	呼吸器内科	12
☐	reticulocyte count	網状赤血球、レチクロ	151
☐	return visit	再診	25
☐	rheumatoid arthritis	関節リウマチ	170
☐	rheumatologist	リウマチ専門医	170, 189

☐	rheumatology	リウマチ科	12
☐	rhinitis	鼻炎	278
☐	root canals	歯根管	286
☐	rotablator	ロータブレーター	144
☐	rotary-chair testing	回転椅子検査	270
☐	rule out	～を除外する	102
☐	runny nose	鼻水	33

S

☐	salve	軟膏	226, 250
☐	sciatica	坐骨神経痛	98
☐	second trimester	妊娠中期（第2期）	234
☐	secondhand smoke	副流煙	118
☐	secrete	分泌する	153
☐	seizure	発作	206
☐	self-exam	自己検診（セルフチェック）	218
☐	self-medicating	自己治療	168
☐	serum	血清	149
☐	sharp pain	激しい痛み	39
☐	short fuse	癇癪	167
☐	shortness of breath	息切れ	34
☐	side effect	副作用	73, 74
☐	silent ischemia	無症候性虚血	204
☐	sinus infection	副鼻腔炎	278
☐	sinus pain	副鼻腔の痛み	35
☐	sinus rhythm	サイナスリズム（洞調律）	132
☐	sinuses	洞、副鼻腔	102, 278
☐	sitz bath	座浴	226
☐	skin allergies	皮膚アレルギー	250
☐	skin tag	スキン・タグ、軟性線維腫	254
☐	skin tumors	できもの	254
☐	sleep study	睡眠検査	124
☐	slow arrhythmia	頻脈性不整脈	135
☐	sore throat	喉の痛み	33
☐	spinal stenosis	脊髄管狭窄症	101
☐	spinal tap	腰椎穿刺	69
☐	spiral CT	スパイラルCT、螺旋CT	243
☐	sprains	捻挫	186
☐	sputum test	喀痰検査	69
☐	stabbing pain	刺すような痛み	39

☐	stay overnight	一晩入院する	82
☐	stenosis	狭窄症	185
☐	stent	ステント	145
☐	stiff neck	首凝り	35, 185
☐	stiff shoulder	肩凝り	185
☐	stomachache	胃痛	35
☐	stool	排泄物	226
☐	stool test	検便	69
☐	stress test	負荷検査	131
☐	stroke	脳卒中	210
☐	syncope	失神	135
☐	swollen	（足が）むくむ	33

T

☐	tender	圧痛のある、触ると痛い	147
☐	tension headache	緊張性[型]頭痛	104
☐	tetanus shot	破傷風の予防注射	193
☐	thermography	サーモグラフィー	69
☐	throbbing pain	ずきずきする痛み	39
☐	thyroid	甲状腺	165, 214, 261
☐	tingling	うずくような痛み	39
☐	tinnitus	耳鳴り	274
☐	tissue under the skin	皮下組織	172
☐	toothache	歯痛	35
☐	tranquilizer	精神安定剤、鎮痛剤	277
☐	transmit	感染する	238
☐	treadmill exercise test	トレッドミル運動負荷検査	122
☐	treatable	治療可能である	125
☐	trichotillomania	抜毛癖	261
☐	tumor marker	腫瘍マーカー	221

U

☐	UC (Ulcerative Colitis)	潰瘍性大腸炎	106
☐	ulcers	胃潰瘍	110
☐	ultrasound	超音波検査	64, 69, 218 230
☐	underweight	体重不足の	234
☐	urethra	尿道	238
☐	urinalysis	尿検査	69, 115
☐	urination	排尿	238
☐	urine output measurements	尿排出量検査	115

☐	urology	泌尿器科	12
☐	uterine cancer screening	子宮がん検査法	69
☐	uterus	子宮	236
☐	UTI (urinary tract infection)	尿路感染症	238

V

☐	vaginal birth	普通分娩	236
☐	vaporizer	気化器	105
☐	vertebra	椎骨、脊椎骨(複数形:vertebrae)	196
☐	vital capacity (VC)	肺活量	123
☐	vitals	バイタルサイン	87, 92
☐	vitamin B-12	ビタミンB12	150

W

☐	wait and see	経過観察	194, 230
☐	wheeze	ゼーゼー息をする	118
☐	white blood cell	白血球	109
☐	white coat hypertension	白衣高血圧	137
☐	work-up	精密検査	103
☐	wounds	傷	190

X

☐	X-ray	レントゲン	64, 69

● 監修者 ●
Barry Blum, MD（バリー・ブラム医学博士）
整形外科医
Alii Health Center (Kailua-Kona, Hawaii)
Kona Comunity Hospital 元院長
West Hawaii Regional Board, Hawaii Health Systems Corporation (HHSC) 元会長

● 著者 ●
Shari J. Berman（バーマン・シャーリー・J）
米国オハイオ州立大学卒。バーモント州School for International Trainingで英語教授法 (TESOL) の修士号を取得。1976年来日後、有限会社ジャパン・ランゲージ・フォーラムを設立し英語教育、教材執筆、翻訳に携わる。2012年4月より弘前大学国際教育センター准教授、2020年4月より同大学大学院医学研究科特任准教授を勤める。主な著書に「医師のための正しく伝わる・必ず返事が来る英文メールの書き方」（ナツメ社）がある。

● 校閲 ●
山名 哲夫 東京山手メディカルセンター（旧 社会保険中央病院）
　　　　　　大腸肛門病センター部長
佐藤 哲観 静岡県立静岡がんセンター 緩和医療科医長
　　　　　　弘前大学医学部附属病院 麻酔科・緩和ケア診療室 元病棟医長

● スタッフ ●
本文デザイン	株式会社シー・レップス
イラスト	富永三紗子
執筆・編集協力	株式会社シー・レップス
	有限会社ジャパン・ランゲージ・フォーラム
録音	一般財団法人英語教育協議会（ELEC）
ナレーター	Howard Colefield　Edith Kayumi
	吉田浩二　春田ゆり
編集担当	遠藤やよい（ナツメ出版企画株式会社）

ナツメ社Webサイト
http://www.natsume.co.jp
書籍の最新情報（正誤情報を含む）はナツメ社Webサイトをご覧ください。

CD付き 正しく診断するための診療英会話

2016年 7月 7日 初版発行
2020年11月10日 第4刷発行

監修者　バリー・ブラム　　　　　　　　　　　　Barry Blum, 2016
著　者　バーマン・シャーリー・J　　　　　　© Shari J. Berman, 2016
発行者　田村正隆

発行所　株式会社ナツメ社
　　　　東京都千代田区神田神保町1-52ナツメ社ビル1F（〒101-0051）
　　　　電話 03 (3291) 1257（代表）　　FAX 03 (3291) 5761
　　　　振替 00130-1-58661
制　作　ナツメ出版企画株式会社
　　　　東京都千代田区神田神保町1-52ナツメ社ビル3F（〒101-0051）
　　　　電話 03 (3295) 3921（代表）
印刷所　ラン印刷社

ISBN978-4-8163-5814-2　　　　　　　　　　　　　　　　Printed in Japan
〈定価はカバーに表示してあります〉〈乱丁・落丁本はお取り替えします〉

本書に関するお問い合わせは、上記、ナツメ出版企画株式会社までお願いいたします。

本書の一部または全部を著作権法で定められている範囲を超え、ナツメ出版企画株式会社に無断で複写、複製、転載、データファイル化することを禁じます。